KAISER PERMANENTE
REGIONAL LABORATORY
10220 S.E. SUNNYSIDE ROAD
CLACKAMAS, OR   97015

Total Quality Management in the Clinical Laboratory

Also available from ASQC Quality Press

How to Lower Health Care Costs by Improving Health Care Quality: Results-Based Continuous Quality Improvement
M. Daniel Sloan

Quality Improvement Handbook for Health Care Professionals
James P. Mozena and Debby L. Anderson

Guidelines for Laboratory Quality Auditing
Donald C. Singer and Ronald P. Upton

Benchmarking: The Search for Industry Best Practices That Lead to Superior Performance
Robert C. Camp

Quality Assurance in Health Care Services
Raandi Schmidt, Judith Trumbo, and Ross Johnson, editors

The Quality Revolution and Health Care
M. Daniel Sloan and Micheal Chmel, M.D.

Total Quality and Productivity Management in Health Care Organizations
Vincent K. Omachonu, Ph.D.

To request a complimentary catalog of publications, call 800-248-1946.

Total Quality Management in the Clinical Laboratory

Doug Hutchison

American Association of Bioanalysts
St. Louis, Missouri

ASQC Quality Press
Milwaukee, Wisconsin

Total Quality Management in the Clinical Laboratory
Doug Hutchison

Library of Congress Cataloging-in-Publication Data

Hutchison, Doug.
    Total quality management in the clinical laboratory / Doug Hutchison
        p. cm.
    Includes bibliographical references and index.
    ISBN 0-87389-252-6 (alk. paper)
    1. Pathological laboratories—Quality control. 2. Total quality management.
  3. Pathological laboratories—Management. I. Title.
    [DNLM: 1. Laboratories—standards. 2. Chemistry, Clinical.
  3. Quality Control. QY 23 H978t 1994]
  RB36.3.Q34H88 1994
  616.07'5'068—dc20
  DNLM/DLC
  for Library of Congress   93-42922
                                            CIP

10 9 8 7 6 5 4 3 2 1

ISBN 0-87389-252-6

Acquisitions Editor: Susan Westergard
Project Editor: Kelley Cardinal
Production Editor: Annette Wall
Marketing Administrator: Mark Olson
Set in Caslon 540 and Gill Sans by Montgomery Media, Inc.
Cover design by Montgomery Media, Inc.
Printed and bound by BookCrafters, Inc.

ASQC Mission: To facilitate continuous improvement and increase customer satisfaction by identifying, communicating, and promoting the use of quality principles, concepts, and technologies; and thereby be recognized throughout the world as the leading authority on, and champion for, quality.

For a free copy of the ASQC Quality Press Publications Catalog, including ASQC membership information, call 800-248-1946.

Printed in the United States of America

 Printed on acid-free recycled paper

 American Association of Bioanalysts
818 Olive Street, Suite 918
St. Louis, Missouri 63101

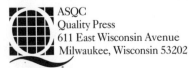 ASQC
Quality Press
611 East Wisconsin Avenue
Milwaukee, Wisconsin 53202

Contents

Figures and Tables

Figures

Tables

Foreword

As consumers lament the terrible state of the health care industry, health care administrators are turning to the concepts and principles of total quality management for badly needed answers. The power base has shifted dramatically from the sellers of health care services to the buyers. The buyers have more choices today than at any other time in history.

Health care laboratories and their affiliated clinical disciplines have increasingly become the focal point for quality improvement and cost containment opportunities. Dr. Doug Hutchison's book *Total Quality Management in the Clinical Laboratory* provides a critical blueprint for understanding and implementing TQM in the clinical laboratory. In a clearly presented format, Dr. Hutchison has examined how the principles of Dr. W. Edwards Deming and Dr. Joseph M. Juran can be applied to the clinical laboratory setting.

Practitioners and academicians alike will find Dr. Hutchison's book invaluable as they chart the course of organizational excellence and competitiveness. The book should prove to be a fine addition to the existing literature on total quality in health care organizations.

Vincent K. Omachonu, Ph.D., P.E.
University of Miami
Institute for the Study of Quality

Preface

This book is written for the people of the clinical lab. While the subject of this book, total quality management (TQM), is indeed a management technique, these pages should prove helpful to those associated with the lab whether they are suppliers, workers, or users of the services. The lab is viewed as a system which has various inputs such as supplies, reagents, and specimens. The lab also has outputs in the form of reports that reflect the quality of the testing operation and the quality of the people who did the testing. This information-generation and delivery process must integrate equally well with both internal and external factors.

The book is written using the principles of W. Edwards Deming and Joseph M. Juran, the two primary contributors to the quality movement in Japan. Their work resulted in Japan's recognized position of distinction with regard to the quality of its products and services.

Although the focus of this book is the clinical lab, the perspective is much broader. Just as there are several types of clinical laboratories, the people of the clinical lab may also have dissimilar backgrounds and responsibilities. Hence I address the TQM principles from the perspective of senior management, middle and line management, the line workers, users, and suppliers. As such, this book is substantially more than a technical exposé. The writing has been deliberately kept descriptive, so that the concepts of TQM can be easily grasped. The perspective is one in which the elements of TQM are described as completely as space allows, so that TQM stands out as an integrated pathway offering perspective on many different aspects of business circumstance.

Following a description of the history and philosophy of TQM, the book proceeds to investigate sources of lab error, the TQM tools that are used to investigate system error, and the design process improvements that enhance reliability. Statistics relating to these operations are reviewed. A detailed and practical approach to deploying TQM in the lab setting is presented. TQM aspects of the Clinical Laboratory Improvement Act of 1988 (CLIA '88), such as process validation, as well as international standards, are reviewed. The book concludes with a review of the Baldrige criteria used in a hospital lab environment. The appendices offer a protocol for writing lab procedures using the CLIA '88 quality assurance program as illustration.

Acknowledgments

I would like to thank John Cramer of American Hydrosurgical Instruments for sharing reference materials with me. My gratitude to Paul Blackinton, formerly of Federal Express for sharing insights gained there. Thanks also to Dr. Jill Swift of the University of Miami School of Engineering for her thoughts on applied statistics.

My appreciation is extended to Kersi Munshi, former senior analyst at Florida Power & Light (FPL) for discussions on policy management. Others at FPL who helped me were Bud Hunter, former senior vice president and now head of Leland Hunter Management Associate; Bill Davis, former manager of end-use technology and research, now of Davis Consulting; and Bill Klein, former vice president of business development at FPL and now head of WMK Enterprises.

Appreciation is extended to Ruth Marrero for sharing data with me on spinal fluid turnaround time. The associated flowchart and Ishikawa diagram are hers as well. Thanks to Orlando Acevedo of Coulter Electronics, my trainer for the ASQC/CQE, and the insights gained into the contributions of Joseph M. Juran to the TQC effort.

It is with gratitude that I acknowledge the helpful role of Dr. Howard Gitlow of the University of Miami Institute for Quality. Dr. Gitlow read parts of the manuscript as well as helped me form many of the understandings I developed relevant to TQM and the role Dr. Deming played in it.

I would like to recognize the contributions of Matt Weinrich of Genzyme who shared some key thoughts with me regarding the role of sales and marketing in the quality effort. Thanks also to Kathy Leedy of the

National Institute of Standards and Technology, and to Jim Sierk of Allied Signal for the excellent training on the Malcolm Baldrige National Quality Award, and to the many examiners who shared their expertise with me.

Thanks to my wife Louise and my children Kurt, Drew, Lynn, and Laurie, who, in their many roles, made this book truly a team effort. Their understanding and support over the past year was integral to its completion.

My gratitude to David Birenbaum and Dr. Mark Birenbaum, long-time friends and administrators of the American Association of Bioanalysts, who underwrote my early efforts in this field.

Thank you all.

1

Introduction to Total Quality Management

THE SCIENTIFIC WAY OF DOING BUSINESS

Plan, Do, Check, Act. With these four words, in 1936, Walter A. Shewhart unknowingly began a quality revolution which rocketed through post-war Japan and now is being embraced by industrial leaders in the United States like a long-lost friend. The remarkable thing about this reformation is that it had to be imported from Japan even though it began in the United States and was introduced to the Japanese by Americans.

The reason these teachings weren't initially adopted in the United States was due to a combination of affairs that included uncritical post-war consumers, economic policies that included planned obsolescence, and the acerbic disposition of the plan's chief promoter, Dr. W. Edwards Deming. The technique became known in Japan as TQC, total quality control, and in the United States as total quality management or TQM. The latter better describes the teachings, because they are, in effect, a management system. While they incorporate quality control techniques, they go much further than quality control.

ORIGINS OF TQM

Total quality management is a technique developed by a small group of American quality professionals and exported to Japan shortly after the end of World War II. One of the chief aspects of TQM is viewing quality from the perspective of the customer or consumer. Before this, companies defined quality as meeting internal specifications. Under TQM, quality is defined by the user. One contributor to early TQM described this as "fitness for use."

TQM is also based on companywide involvement in quality goals. Quality is no longer a specialist's role limited to a few inspectors or quality control people. For TQM to work it must have commitment from the top management through all levels of the operation. This includes not just the technical component of the plant, but sales, marketing, facilities, customer service, financial, and staff positions as well. Under TQM, quality is everyone's job.

An additional feature of TQM is the use of statistical process control (SPC) or the use of statistical techniques to analyze processes or systems. Unforseen variation in processes is the cause of error, and the established techniques of TQM are used to reduce error to a minimum level.

TQM is not just one more new management paradigm. TQM brought Japan, a nation with a reputation for poor-quality consumer goods, from the devastation of the post-war era to its current position of prominence both in manufacturing and in the service industries. TQM is proven. It worked not only in Japan, but works in this country in U.S. plants with U.S. workers.

There is a check cycle in TQM. This is a review provision which requires that process change and improvement be monitored. In effect, it foolproofs management performance by making certain that what is actually being delivered is what the management strategy intended.

There were a handful of key players in the early days of the Japanese industrial rebirth, and foremost among them was W. Edwards Deming. Deming, a physicist who trained under U.S. quality expert Walter A. Shewhart, had tried repeatedly to get his quality concepts accepted in U.S. industry. In the heady post-war economy the timing was not right, and Deming was characterized as "somewhat of a crank."[1] He joined the U.S. Census Bureau and in that role visited Japan in 1946 and 1948. He began to get a following there and made the acquaintance of a key figure in Japanese industry, Ichiro Ishikawa.

Ishikawa, head of the Keidanren, an influential Japanese business society, used his authority to invite 35 of the foremost business leaders to hear Deming speak on his ideas. General Douglas MacArthur had said that the Japanese could have unions, and this group had founded the Union of Japanese Scientists and Engineers (JUSE). JUSE took Deming's advice to heart and the Japanese TQC story began to unfold (see Table 1.1 and Figure 1.1).

Table 1.1: Important dates in the development of TQM.

1945	The Union of Japanese Scientists and Engineers (JUSE) is formed.
1946	The American Society for Quality Control (ASQC) is formed. George Edwards is elected its first president.
1950	Deming addresses JUSE.
1951	The Deming Prize is established.
1954	Juran is invited to speak to JUSE.
1957	Walter A. Shewhart visits Japan.
1962	QC circle activities begin.
1969	First International Society of QC meeting is held in Tokyo.
1971	Kaoru Ishikawa wins ASQC Grant Award.
1974	QC Symposium for Service Industry is coordinated by Juran.
1976	Yoshio Kendo wins ASQC Grant Award.
1980	Thirty-five countries now using QC circles.
1982	Kaoru Ishikawa wins ASQC's Shewhart medal.
1985	Ishikawa's *What Is Total Quality Control—The Japanese Way* is released in English.
1987	The Malcolm Baldrige National Quality Award is introduced in the United States.
1988	First winners of the Baldrige Award are Motorola, Westinghouse's Nuclear Fuel Division, and Globe Metallurgical in the small business category.
1989	Florida Power & Light is the first U.S. company to win the Deming Prize.

W. Edwards Deming, Ph.D., author of *Out of the Crisis*, is credited by the Japanese for being key to their post-war industrial quality efforts. Born in 1900, Deming graduated from Yale in 1927 with a doctorate in mathematical physics. Japan named the Deming Prize after him. This award is Japan's second most prestigious business award, the most prestigious being the Japan Prize. To challenge for the latter, the business must have won the Deming Prize during the previous five years. The Japan Prize would have been named after Dr. Juran, but he declined the honor. Deming is widely regarded as bringing SPC and the concept of special- and common-cause variation to the Japanese and to the operator level of understanding. Deming was nominated for the Nobel Prize in Economics in 1992.

Joseph M. Juran, BSEE, J.D., author of *Managerial Breakthrough* and *Juran's Quality Control Handbook*, is also considered a major architect of Japan's industrial rebirth in the early 1950s. He is most recognized for bringing a management theory to the Japanese that included the concept of process ownership by supervision and the role of management in handling special- and common-cause variation.

Walter A. Shewhart, Ph.D., a mathematical physicist like Deming, was a mentor of Deming's and lists contributions to industrial quality control dating to the 1920s and 1930s. A version of the Shewhart control chart is used in the clinical lab for charting instrument performance on QC samples and for determining run reliability.

George Edwards, Ph.D., a colleague of Shewhart, was instrumental in forming the American Society for Quality Control (ASQC). He was elected its first president in 1946. This organization has assumed a key role in disseminating TQM to U.S. industries, and currently administers the Malcom Baldrige National Quality Award, the most prestigious U.S. business award named after the former secretary of commerce.

Armand Feigenbaum, a quality management expert in the United States, published the book *Total Quality Control* in the 1960s. The Japanese liked the term and took it back with them to identify their own efforts.

Howard Gitlow, Ph.D. in applied statistics, is director of the Institute for the Study of Quality at the University of Miami. He is the author of several books including *Planning for Quality Productivity and Competitive Position*. Gitlow was a student of Deming's at New York University.

Figure 1.1: Key figures in TQM.

Joseph M. Juran, another U.S. quality expert who trained as an engineer, went to Japan and addressed JUSE in 1954. He published the first edition of *Juran's Quality Control Handbook* the following year. The latest edition (1988) runs nearly 1800 pages. Juran's major contributions included defining the role of management in TQM terms. He saw managers as process improvement coordinators. Deming, meanwhile, brought applied statistics to the level of line operations with the subsequent evolution of SPC in Japan.

Japan named a prestigious quality award in honor of Dr. W. Edwards Deming. The Deming Prize has been a coveted award in Japan since 1951. In the 1970s Professor Kondo of JUSE approached Dr. Juran to establish an even grander award to be named after him. Juran demurred, and so the Japanese conceived of the Japan Prize awarded to the best performer selected from Deming Prize winners during the past five years. In 1985 the Deming Prize was opened up to companies outside of Japan and the first non-Japanese company to win the award was Florida Power & Light (FPL). It used techniques developed by Joseph M. Juran and W. Edwards Deming; however, since it had considerable assistance from the Japanese, FPL is best characterized as a Japanese TQC company.

ADAPTING JAPANESE TQC FOR WESTERN MANAGERS

If there were something special about the Japanese makeup that predisposes it to TQC, something that made TQC inapplicable to western management, a lot of time would be wasted trying to learn it. It would be far better not to take this wrong turn and instead to continue to develop a new western management style. In a sense, that is what is going on, but the new style has deep roots in TQC as well as in the developing philosophies expressed by Deming, Juran, and other TQC principals. Before getting too involved in a management style which may be impossible to adapt to western ways, it is certainly logical to ask if TQC is for the Japanese only or if it can be adapted to western work societies.

Many people have speculated on the nature of Japanese culture versus that of the United States. One aspect of the Japanese culture on which there is agreement is that the Japanese are a homogeneous group; that is, Japanese are all from Japan (or nearby), whereas Americans are almost all from somewhere other than America. In addition to ethnic diversity, there are also many religions and races in the United States that do not exist in Japan.

In theory, this should make western workers more individualistic and less able to do the group interplay required for good cross-functional interaction. In fact, it is easy to get agreement that the Japanese are better than westerners are at group business activities. Hiroshi Osada of Asahi, a company characterized as the Japanese DuPont, recently addressed the issue of Japanese homogeneity by saying, "We may all look the same to you, but we think quite differently." He went on to elaborate about the tumultuous feelings which violently split the country over the issue of participating in Desert Shield.

It was once suggested that Deming management would be an easier sell if it had been introduced to Poland or Italy and made it a world leader in commerce. On the contrary, the Europeans have a tradition of craftsmanship which dates back to the Middle Ages. The French, with caves such as Lascaux and others on the Franco-Cantabrian Plain, point with pride to commerce reaching far back into prehistory.

Japan, on the other hand, had a reputation for the worst consumer goods in the world prior to World War II. For many years *Made in Japan* was a synonym for poor-quality merchandise. Not until 1964 did Nissan, the first winner of the Deming Prize, introduce its first car here. It was called Datsun so that the illustrious name of the parent company wouldn't be disgraced should the car not be accepted. This was a very tentative start. Now, 25 years later, Japanese cars are recognized for their quality just as many other consumer products made in Japan.

Deming told the Japanese in a 1950 address, "Follow me and in 10 years the West will be asking for economic protection from you." This is the business equivalent of Babe Ruth pointing to the left field wall before swatting one out.

Some popular management articles still unwittingly foster the belief that the Japanese have achieved their position by slogan chanting, fanatic devotion to the company way, and inhuman concentration. These characteristics were as much part of the Japanese ethic in the old days, the days of unreliable Japanese products, as they are now. Other things clearly are responsible for quality under the new systems of management.

THE PDCA CYCLE

PDCA stands for Plan, Do, Check, and Act. The PDCA cycle is a visual representation of the scientific method as originally used by Walter A. Shewhart. The circular representation of the four steps is meant to depict the continual nature of the process (see Figure 1.2). Whereas the scientific method prescribes establishing a working hypothesis, or theorem, followed

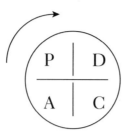

Figure 1.2: The PDCA cycle. The PDCA cycle was originally conceived by Walter A. Shewhart and later introduced to the Japanese by Dr. W. Edwards Deming. The Japanese refer to it as the Deming cycle or Deming wheel. Deming originally introduced it as a way of conceptually linking customer requirements to engineering design.

As the wheel evolved it came to represent the continuous notion of process improvement. When a new process is introduced, it has its roots in the planning (P) process. This is followed by a limited trial of the process as represented by the do (D) quadrant. Following limited deployment, the process is evaluated using the check (C) cycle to see if the process needs modification before proceeding to full deployment, the act (A) cycle. The process is repeated in keeping with company resources and priorities.

by an investigational stage to verify the hypothesis, the PDCA cycle represents these as the planning stage followed by a do stage. The do stage is implementing the results of the planning stage on a limited basis.

In the scientific method, if the theorem is verified repeatedly over time, then it may become law. In the PDCA cycle, if the results of the limited deployment look good in the check cycle review, then a wider deployment is done as portrayed by the act quadrant. Inherent in the act quadrant is a continual internal check process which monitors progress and may lead into the next plan component.

In this same way, Newton's law of gravitation, established and accepted over time, became part of the general theory of relativity as proposed by Einstein. As the wheel continues to turn, both these ideas may someday become part of something much more grand. Whereas the scientific method applies to obtaining knowledge for the sake of knowing, TQM is deployed consistent with the concept of diminishing returns reflected by quality costs. TQM is not a headlong quest for quality at the expense of everything else. The keys to rational TQM deployment are both prioritization and sound resource allocation.

The PDCA cycle is used to manage change in the laboratory, as well as in any business setting. Any process change first goes through a planning stage, followed by limited deployment, followed by an evaluation of how the limited application of the change is doing, followed by modification (if needed), and then full-scale deployment. The Japanese use the expression "how many times did you turn the wheel?" to assess how detailed the process change or improvement was. The component steps of how this is done, and the TQM tools which are used in each of the steps, are discussed in detail in subsequent chapters.

DEMING'S 14 POINTS

These management guidelines were published in 1986 in Deming's book *Out of the Crisis*. They have caused some confusion because people thought that they were, in essence, Japanese TQC summarized by the man who had given the concept to the Japanese. While the 14 points were indeed the crystallization of Deming's ideas to that point, they are relatively unknown in Japan. At this writing, *Out of the Crisis* has not been translated into Japanese. It is critical to understand what is Japanese TQC because it is what has brought business success to the Japanese.

The 14 points provide the architecture for much of the TQM efforts in this country, and with good reason. They are culturally inclined to U.S. business outlook, and they are a modern encapsulation of Deming's thoughts. A cursory look at the highlights of the 14 points is worthwhile simply to show the differences in these guidelines from those of Japanese TQC (see Table 1.2).

Many of these points, as written, are totally unacceptable to the Japanese character. By using terms such as *drive out, cease dependence on*, and *eliminate slogans, quotas*, Deming adopts a phraseology not in keeping with Japanese construction. These are terms simply too dictatorially negative. For acceptance in Japan they need to be rewritten in keeping with the Japanese diplomatic mode of expression. For this country, however, the phraseology is obviously no problem. The following is a review of the 14 points from a Japanese TQC perspective.

Points 1 and 2: These are about adopting the new philosophy and building in constancy of purpose. These are given as fundamental to the Japanese effort as is point 3, incorporating system design for quality rather than end-process inspection. This correlates with point 10 on eliminating slogans. The objective is to design systems to achieve the aims which the slogans exhort.

Point 4: In the United States, there is a serious effort to develop a vendor relationship which rewards vendors for their quality efforts. This has not,

Table 1.2: A theory for management—Deming's 14 points.

1. Create constancy of purpose toward improvement of product and service, with the aim of becoming competitive and to stay in business and to provide jobs.

2. Adopt the new philosophy. We are in a new economic age. Western management must awaken to the challenge, must learn its responsibilities, and take on leadership for change.

3. Cease dependence on inspection to achieve quality. Eliminate the need for inspection on a mass basis by building quality into the product in the first place.

4. End the practice of awarding business on price tag. Instead, minimize total cost. Move toward a single supplier for any one item, on a long-term relationship of loyalty and trust.

5. Improve constantly and forever the system of production and service, to improve the quality and productivity, and thus constantly decrease costs.

6. Institute training on the job.

7. Institute leadership (see point 12). The aim of leadership should be to help people, machines, and gadgets do a better job. Leadership of management is in need of an overhaul, as well as leadership of production workers.

8. Drive out fear, so that everyone may work effectively for the company.

9. Break down barriers between departments. People in research, design, sales, and production must work as a team, to foresee problems of production and use that may be encountered with the product or service.

10. Eliminate slogans, exhortations, and targets for the work force that ask for zero defects and new levels of productivity.

11a. Eliminate work standards (quotas) on the factory floor. Replace standards with leadership.

11b. Eliminate management by objective. Eliminate management by numbers and numerical goals. Replace with leadership.

12a. Remove barriers that rob hourly workers of their right to pride of workmanship. The responsibility of supervisors must be changed from sheer numbers to quality.

continued

Table 1.2: *continued*

12b. Remove barriers that rob people in managment and engineering of their right to pride of workmanship. This means, among other things, abolishment of the annual raise or merit rating and of management by objective and management by the numbers.

13. Institute a vigorous program of education and self-improvement.

14. Put everybody in the company to work to accomplish the transformation. The transformation is everybody's job.

---

to my knowledge, had any impact on the way lab clients interact with the lab. This is critical to the success of quality efforts in labs. Much of the business relationship that the lab has with clinical accounts is predicated on reimbursement policies installed by government or insurance practices. These are fiscal policies and generally leave no room for the recognition of quality work. This must change. Currently lab business is awarded pretty much on the basis of price tag alone.

Point 5: The process of continual improvement is central to Japanese TQM teaching. The quality effort is a never-ending process.

Points 6 and 13: On-the-job training, internal and external formal education, and job-related guidance are critical to the success of TQC.

Point 7: This point as well as number 12 delve into the leader's role in TQM. Deming believes that a leader (supervisor or director) derives his or her power to lead from three sources: (1) positional or situational components; (2) knowledge; and (3) charisma. People will listen to the boss (positional) or a mugger with a gun (situational). The wise executive stresses knowledge and charisma. There is undoubtedly a link between charisma and position if you think for a minute of Ronald Reagan as Hollywood actor or as president of the United States. Same man, very different charisma.

Point 8: If there is one common denominator to all U.S. management practices, it has got to be fear. Shape up or ship out. In Japan, the deal is deliver what is asked and you have a lifetime job. The downside to this is that if you don't deliver and get asked to leave, outside employment chances are pretty dim.

Points 9 and 12: Removing barriers to communication and to other aspects of implementing TQC must be done early in the deployment of this management program. Japanese managers who have implemented TQC continually refer to barriers to progress which had to be surmounted in order for TQC to progress. Also in point 12 is perhaps the most controversial of Deming's points, the elimination of the annual raise tied to achievement of goals. This is partially tied to the depth with which management by objective is ingrained here. U.S. executives also feel they may be exposing themselves to liability if some sort of score is not kept on who does good and who doesn't. The records need to be there in case the Labor Department comes calling.

Point 14: From the TQM standpoint, quality is indeed everyone's business as compared to earlier times when it was the domain of the quality specialist. TQM only becomes a way of life when it does, in fact, permeate all areas of the business function.

REDEFINING QUALITY

The new definition of quality can best be understood by reflecting on the current definition of quality. As it presently stands quality is defined as doing what the boss wants—right away. This is also a customer-oriented definition of quality; in other words, doing what the customer wants, but the boss is the customer. This is perfectly reasonable from the employee's point of view because the boss sets goals, measures progress, and delivers rewards. So currently, as shown in Figure 1.3, top management is the primary customer, middle management is next, line management follows, and lastly, comes the lowly consumer. This results in a product-out versus a market-in way of doing business. In other words, the entire business focus is on internal priorities rather than consumer interests.

Fig 1.3 shows symbolically how the new paradigm inverts the pyramid and shifts the focus by having the consumer define quality priorities. Integrating the consumer's views into the business system is a highly structured system within TQM. If it were not, then anarchy would result. Inverting the pyramid doesn't mean that no one runs the company anymore. What it means is that the direction of company policies is now partly dictated by the customer's views. This then calls for an organized way of sampling customer requirements. In addition, the consumer's views must be integrated into the company's operation in terms of rational goals based on these needs, and internal systems and processes designed to address these needs. As this is done, the original structure continues in force, but now the focus is not on doing what the boss arbitrarily or whimsically may indicate, but on the continual smooth operation of systems designed to address consumer-identified priorities.

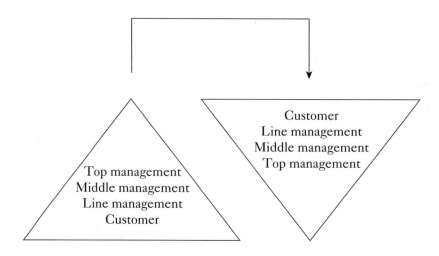

Figure 1.3: Inverting the pyramid. TQM inverts the management pyramid so that the customer's views become paramount in determining what the quality priorities are. The customer can be the end user of the product or service, that is, the consumer, or the customer can be the end user of an internal process. The latter is referred to as an internal customer.

It is worthwhile to more carefully define a few of the terms in the previous paragraph. The *consumer* is the overall end user of the business output. If the laboratory generates reports, then the ultimate user of the reports is the consumer, and this can be the physician, the patient, the contractor, or whomever. Within the laboratory there are many systems which have input and output, or in other words, they have a supplier and a customer. For instance, the front end of a lab usually has an area in which specimens are received, divided, and labeled for positive identification and work lists are prepared and forwarded to the work areas with the samples. This is broadly described as accessioning, and the customers in this case are the bench techs whose needs must be integrated into the work list/specimen-delivery system. These people are known as *internal customers*. The processes described for market-in integration of the consumer's voice are equally valid for the integration of the internal customer's voice into the internal system.

The words *system* and *process* are used interchangeably. A process or system has a supplier (or raw material) and a customer or consumer. Another view is that a system has an input and an output. Productivity is broadly measured as output over input, and output is frequently measured per unit of some kind—per individual or dollar invested for instance. The system will be examined in excruciating detail at various points later, and the reason is twofold. First, using the system for the focus of managerial effort is unique to TQM, and second, getting managers to understand this system focus, as opposed to the pursuit of goals, is a very difficult reorientation.

Lastly, the word *goal* is not often mentioned in a TQM article without some sort of qualifying word. For instance, Deming never uses the word and insists on focusing on the process and letting the goals obtain naturally as a result of the process optimization. His view is that goal setting may result in too low an expectation, whereas focusing on the process will maximize the process output. Thus, users could be pleasantly surprised by exceeding the mark. On the other hand, Gitlow, a Deming adherent, uses the term *rational goals* to identify goals that are set in keeping with the market-in process. To quote Gitlow, "You can't introduce Deming management to top executives by telling them that everything they have ever done is wrong and expect them to say 'Oh thank you master, tell me where we have gone wrong.'" Deming, of course, does this at virtually every opportunity, but Deming wants to break the back of the old management system. Gitlow's approach is both more diplomatic and in keeping with Japanese TQC, which routinely establishes goals as part of the quality effort. It is important to emphasize, however, that these goals are quite different than the current irrational goals used in business that are generally based on wishes which the system may not be able to deliver and which no one except the boss may view as important. The rational goals are customer-derived and integrated into the business in a very special way. This will be explored in detail later.

The traditional view of quality had been "conformance to specifications." In other words, prior to TQC, businesses defined their best quality efforts as meeting specifications which had been set by the business. This is the product-out perspective and is beset by certain limitations. First, the specifications were routinely set to reflect what the company viewed as optimum without regard for the user's view of the product, and second, it did not take into account service-systems integration in which the output of one service served as the input for the next. There was no focus on the alignment of services as process components.

A step along the evolutionary trail of quality was made by Juran who defined quality as "fitness for use." This view reoriented the company's focus to concentrate on the customer's view of quality and converted companies who were product-out into market-in companies. Since the customer could also be viewed as internal or external, this definition was suitable for

aligning the process components so that the service users were able to provide feedback to their suppliers, so that the suppliers could align their specifications to retain the user's fitness for use.

Later, Philip Crosby, a U.S. quality expert, similarly defined quality
by calling it "conformance to customer requirements" which he subsequently modified to read "conformance to *reasonable* customer requirements." Crosby defined this as the *zero-defect goal.* If the product met the
customer requirements it was then, in all respects, free from defects. These
definitions of quality are self-limiting, and it took further insight to show
just why.

Another authority, Genichi Taguchi, defines quality in an inverse
sense as "the minimal loss to society after shipment (or rendering of service)." Taguchi incorporates the market-in view by appointing society (or
the customer) as the final arbiter, but he introduces something quite new,
and this is the concept of a minimum. He implies that the customer's view
of quality centers around some optimum value and that the process delivery
can vary in a continuous way around that value.

This refocuses the service provider not to meet specifications, as suggested by Juran and Crosby, but to think in terms of integrating processes.
Here, each process component feeds another, and the goal is to center each
process around an optimal value and to continually improve the process
delivery until all components integrate as well as possible with each other.

Since the concept of a minimum loss immediately suggests to mathematicians a point where the first derivative of the descriptive function
equals zero, Taguchi implemented his now-famous loss function in which
he used a parabolic function to describe qualitatively how deviation from
optimal values would affect process performance. This is explored in more
detail in the section on profound knowledge.

Deming defines service quality as "predictable, uniform, and
dependable at low cost, suitable to the market." Once again the market-in
perspective is emphasized, and when combined with his statement that
"the customer never invented anything," Deming provides a formula
encompassing innovation as well. Both are necessary for continuing a company's viability and competitive position.

To more fully appreciate the dimension of TQM, it is helpful to compare it to other management systems. Figure 1.4 shows some of the major
management philosophies over the past 50 years, and the subsequent sections discuss how these ideologies contrast with TQM.

I will try to be particulary careful to characterize what is Deming's, what is Juran's, what is Japanese TQC, and what isn't. This is very important, because, logically, it makes sense to buy into the Japanese method simply because it has been proven to work. Anything else, while perhaps perfectly valid in certain settings, is part of something else, and only critical inspection can reveal whether it is theory, hypothesis, or something more substantial. There are also many western managers who have a perfectly justified skepticism of another management fad, and unless well understood and carefully applied, attempts to deploy TQM by the inexperienced can result in just another botched attempt to run things right.

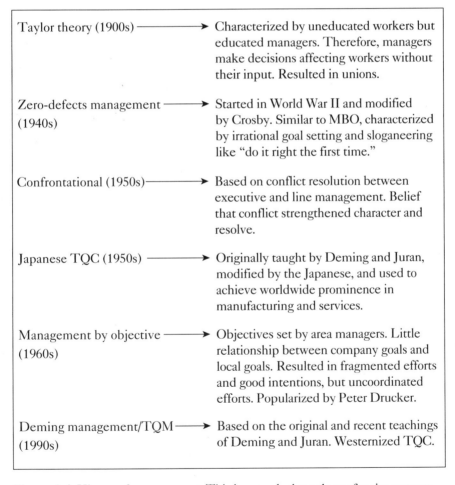

Taylor theory (1900s) ⟶	Characterized by uneducated workers but educated managers. Therefore, managers make decisions affecting workers without their input. Resulted in unions.
Zero-defects management (1940s) ⟶	Started in World War II and modified by Crosby. Similar to MBO, characterized by irrational goal setting and sloganeering like "do it right the first time."
Confrontational (1950s) ⟶	Based on conflict resolution between executive and line management. Belief that conflict strengthened character and resolve.
Japanese TQC (1950s) ⟶	Originally taught by Deming and Juran, modified by the Japanese, and used to achieve worldwide prominence in manufacturing and services.
Management by objective (1960s) ⟶	Objectives set by area managers. Little relationship between company goals and local goals. Resulted in fragmented efforts and good intentions, but uncoordinated efforts. Popularized by Peter Drucker.
Deming management/TQM (1990s) ⟶	Based on the original and recent teachings of Deming and Juran. Westernized TQC.

Figure 1.4: History of management. This is a rough chronology of major management philosophies from Taylor's original conception to the present day. By no means all inclusive, each major style is briefly characterized.

MANAGEMENT BY POLICY AND MANAGEMENT BY OBJECTIVE

The most popular management technique in the United States over the past 10 years has been management by objective (MBO). Popularized by Peter Drucker, MBO, as originally conceived, portrayed corporate objectives being deployed throughout the working ranks, and departmental goals being generated in response to these intents. Through no fault of Drucker's, MBO didn't work like that, and goals were generated by managers on an ad hoc basis and used to promote provincial gain. The objectives became regionalized and subject to local interpretation so that short-term goals became more a reflection of a given manager's viewpoint than bearing any relationship to long-range corporate objectives.

Deming's 11th and 12th points repeatedly say to eliminate management by objective. Table 1.3 contrasts management by objective (MBO) and management by policy (MBP).

MBP, known in Japan as *hoshin kanri*, begins with a top-level policy design which is spread downward by a method of policy deployment. The importance of this top-level support was emphasized in a recent seminar I attended on Japanese TQC. There were about 200 people in a room reviewing a TQM concept, and a woman in the back introduced herself as a

Table 1.3: MBO versus MBP.

MBO	*MBP*
Getting things done through people. People are tools.	Getting things done with people. People are part of the system.
Results oriented.	Policy oriented.
Objectives by manager/employee.	Objectives consistent throughout organization.
Based on external motivation.	Based on internal motivation.
Employees left to own devices to achieve goals.	Means are provided (enablement).
Periodic review of compliance.	Diagnostic review with help (empowerment).

facilitator who worked with a large group of engineers. She was having difficulty getting them to record the needed documentation. While she was musing over what path to take, Dr. Howard Gitlow, of the University of Miami Institute for the Study of Quality, asked her if the company president had bought into TQM. She replied, "No, and neither has the executive vice-president, and . . ."

Gitlow interrupted and said, "There's your problem. Until they do, don't even bother to try."

ZERO-DEFECTS MANAGEMENT

Zero-defects management dates back to World War II. An industrial campaign promoted zero defects. Most manufacturing programs didn't work, and the few that did work, didn't do so as a result of rally-around-the-flag types of advice. Deming's point 10 urges managers to "eliminate slogans . . . asking for zero defects."

Recently, zero-defects management has been popularized by Philip Crosby in a book with the engaging title *Quality Is Free*. In capsule form, zero-defects management asks that zero-defect goals be instituted. Zero-defect goals do not mean that there are no defects. The zero-defect goal is a set of allowable limits on a process that must be met at all times. This is like the two-standard deviation quality control charts in the lab. The zero-defect goal is to be within these limits at all times to release a run.

This is also referred to as goalpost orientation or zero-defect thinking. It is at odds with Deming management from the standpoint that it doesn't encompass continual improvement into the system. In addition, zero-defect thinking doesn't account for a lack of fit between the process delivery and the customer need. For instance, if the lab analytical system delivered glucose values at ± 20 percent reliably, this would be the zero-defect goal, but it wouldn't be good enough for the physician to diagnose incipient diabetes. This is quantified by the Taguchi loss function which reflects the distance away a process is from delivering nominal performance.

There is an additional component to Crosby's zero-defect system which is expressed in the July 1991 *Quality Digest* article entitled "Whatever Happened to Zero Defects?" The argument purports that if an individual is expected to find his or her way home correctly every day, why not expect that person to perform at this perfect level in the job setting?

This won't work in the laboratory due to the impact associated with making an error. In the commuter example, a mistake results in the subject going into the wrong house. In a lab setting, the mistake can cost a life or many lives.

The worst scenario is when an unwitting manager sets a zero-defect goal at no mistakes for a system delivering an output subject to statistical variation. It can't be done. Setting a performance limit at zero defects simply breeds cynicism in the employees. They know intuitively that they aren't perfect even though they may wish that they could be. Having an administrative goal set at perfection of individual performance simply displays human inadequacies in a harsher light. This is particularly true if the zero-defect goal has been set by management without providing the means to obtain the goal. Table 1.4 contrasts key features of zero-defect management and TQM.

SELLING TQM

TQM is necessary because U.S. companies and businesses face many external and internal pressures. Some of these are in the form of increased regulatory burden. The Clinical Laboratory Improvement Act of 1988 (CLIA '88) has just issued new regulations, and labs, for the first time, are under specific Occupational Safety and Health Administration (OSHA) regulations. Other pressures faced are in the form of increased competition for good employees. Once the TQM working environment becomes widely known, new graduates will certainly opt for it as opposed to anything else. There is increased competition in the marketplace, and TQM helps in meeting these challenges. Despite all of this, it may become necessary to convince U.S. management that TQM is the management philosophy that will help it stay competitive and enhance productivity.

Table 1.4: Zero-defects management versus TQM.

Zero defects	TQM
Do it right the first time.	Design a system insensitive to variation.
Zero defects defined as meeting internal specifications every time.	Quality defined as optimizing system output around customer needs.

Deming never makes an attempt to sell TQM in the classical sense. He makes a point of only going into companies to which he has been invited. Just as the first step to curing an illness is the recognition that one is sick, so Deming feels the first step to curing the maladies of conventional management is company recognition that its system needs an overhaul.

Dr. Noriaki Kano, who was one of the key players in the conversion of FPL to Japanese TQM, was viewed as quite brutal by Dr. Howard Gitlow when they consulted there together. Gitlow is director of the Quality Institute at the University of Miami. Kano badgered FPL managers repeatedly during his early visits. The Japanese have a word for this confrontational style of interrogation in which they square off in front of a manager and ask direct probing questions which, for the most part, are unanswerable. If the managers understand Japanese TQC they could handle these, but early on, no one did. For instance, FPL managers were asked, "What do you do?" Typical replies would include a litany of daily functions which included meetings, phone calls, training sessions, and so on. Kano would just repeat, "But what do you do?"

What he eventually got across was Juran's belief that managers were process owners and improvers. In other words, Kano wanted to hear what systems were under the direction of the managers, what they had done and were doing to improve the systems, and what controls had been put in place to maintain the systems at a consistently high level.

Now Kano could have explained this, but he chose to be brutal, insulting, and intimidating. Later, as things progressed and he became gradually more humane, Kano explained to Gitlow that he had been breaking the back of the existing system of management.

Deming uses this same approach. He is a master of overstatement and hyperbole. Again, he feels that this is necessary to bring western management to its senses. Deming has characterized his teachings as a new religion. One of the characteristics of a successful new religion is its ability to encompass old beliefs and enfold the brethren of the old order into the new.

Deming's confrontational approach may be a reflection of his early experience with U.S. managers, in which they essentially ignored him and forced him to teach his principles in Japan rather than his native country. For instance, Deming has characterized U.S. management as having a "negative scrap value." This is like having an old refrigerator you want to sell, and finding that you have to pay someone cash to cart it away. Executives accustomed to patronage dislike being depicted like this.

Although TQM must begin with top-level support and endorsement, even senior management is not immune to selling TQM. They still must present to the board a long-range view bringing quality goals into the same prominence as fiscal. Given the makeup of most of today's boards, this is not an easy sell.

Halberstam, in *The Reckoning* comments on Deming's view as follows, "The Japanese manager's roots were in science or engineering as were those of the board that judged him, while the American manager came from a business or law school, as did the board that judged *him*."[2]

In this regard, the lab has uncommonly talented people and this makes the introduction of Deming management easy and its appeal widespread. Most lab managers have a technical background, and the level of technical expertise of the staff is exceptional as well. Deming, Juran, and Shewhart were all technical specialists who brought applied statistics and scientific management to the line level. Laboratory workers are easily able to understand and make use of the Deming methods. This attribute stems from their training and education and probably from the natural inclination which brought them to the laboratory field in the first place.

HOW TQM INCREASES PRODUCTIVITY

TQM has numerous engaging features, particularly the humanistic characteristics, so that it may appeal to the philanthropic manager. As such, it is easy to lose sight of the features that make TQM important in the intense competitive arena of the workplace. Deming says that he hopes the greediest, most self-serving corporate executives hear about his management technique, because it puts money in their pockets. It does this by increasing the company's productivity. In short, the company does more, and it does it more efficiently.

Another way of viewing the costs of doing business is to divide them into fixed and variable costs. In brief, the fixed costs are those associated with the overall running of the business. These are the costs which exist independent of whether a product or service is being produced. Rent is a good example. The rent payment is indifferent to the activities of the workplace, and it must be paid whether anyone is doing anything, or whether or not anyone is even at work. Most businesses are centered around an eight-hour daylight productivity period. Labs are generally more efficient than this and spread the resources over a longer work period. The sum of all the fixed costs can be called overhead and must be borne more or less equally by all activities.

The variable costs are those associated with a given product or service. For instance, every time a test is run, there is an associated reagent cost, a labor cost, perhaps an instrument cost, and other costs directly associated with the project. The more work that is done, the more money that must be expended to support the effort. These are the variable costs. The sum of the fixed and variable costs are the total costs. This figure is the one which must be met to break even.

Figure 1.5 shows the relationship of costs and sales dollars and the break-even point. Deming management makes the break-even point more easily reached by virtue of two different effects. First, it increases sales by the use of quality function deployment, or a market-in versus a product-out way of doing business. This is fully discussed in chapter 5. Secondly, it decreases costs by streamlining and integrating processes and decreasing the labor component of the variable costs. Other costs are also targets of the procedure and are amenable to more efficient use of space and time, which essentially reduces the apportionment of the fixed cost to the project unit.

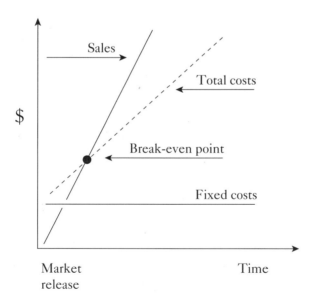

Figure 1.5: Cost of sales. This shows the relationship of cost of sales to business expenses. Total costs are the sum of fixed and variable costs. The break-even point is that sales figure which equals the total cost.

In summary, TQM increases sales and decreases costs, both fixed and variable. This sounds simple, but it is the fundamental reason behind the practicality of Deming management.

QUALITY COSTS

One of the key goals in deploying TQM is raising quality issues to the same prominence as financial issues. Companies are in business to make money for owners and stockholders, not to pursue some other abstract goal. Thus, the quality effort must be designed in keeping with sound financial principles. The TQM effort is designed to clearly document process improvement. It can only do this in a cost-effective manner if the associated cost accounting is done too.

Juran divides quality costs into three broad categories: appraisal, prevention, and failure. Appraisal costs are encountered most commonly in the lab. These include certification of reagents and controls; maintenance costs for instrumentation; calibration of any measurement system, including cost of calibration materials and the overhead associated with the instrument; periodic checks on volumetric equipment; materials and services used in this effort; incoming quality control testing and release of reagents; test kits; and other materials. Prevention costs include process improvement and the associated quality planning, company-subsidized training and education, and correlating, analyzing, and reporting the collected quality data.

The example of pH measurement may help clarify things. If pH is being used to qualify a reagent or solution for production use, then the entire process, pH meter, its maintenance and calibration, and overhead become a quality appraisal cost. On the other hand, if the pH is being measured on a body fluid prior to generating a patient report, then only the instrument preventive maintenance, calibration, and other appraisal costs become assigned to quality. The remaining costs of the instrument, overhead, and salary component of the assay are production costs.

The point is not to make laboratorians experts in cost accounting. Rather, the point is to establish a framework of related quality costs which will help verify what these are, and whether the quality costs are appropriate.

Philip Crosby's expression "quality is free" is based on balancing prevention and appraisal costs against failure costs.[3] Failure costs in a product industry relate to external costs such as warranties and replacing goods and internal costs such as scrap and rework. In the lab industry these costs are reflected internally in customer-service functions and no-charge retesting, and externally as lost accounts or customer dissatisfaction which may result in bad publicity. Costs associated with civil lawsuits for alleged nonperformance may be viewed in this category also.

Figure 1.6 shows the relationship between the three major cost categories—failure costs, process improvement costs, and quality costs. The principle is that increasing prevention quality expenditures will decrease failure costs. This is the central teaching of Japanese TQC and is emphasized in Deming's teaching which advises to "cease reliance on inspection and final test." Process design in keeping with quality goals is the key. The process design must be such as to convey quality to the testing service at each step of the assay trail, from specimen acquisition through reporting.

The aim is to balance quality costs just to the right of the minimum of the sum of the failure and appraisal costs. Too far to the right of this point is the zone of perfectionism in which quality costs can exceed profits. This is not necessarily bad economics if the business is making its initial efforts at a quality reorganization, and this is viewed as an investment in the future. In addition, quality costs can be deducted as a business expense whereas lost sales opportunities due to a poor-quality performance or image is an intangible which the IRS doesn't recognize.

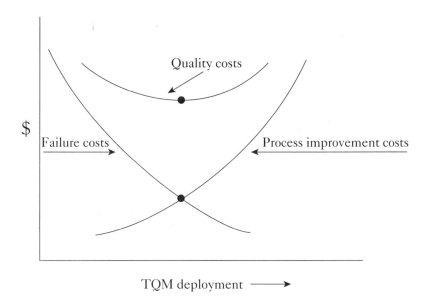

Figure 1.6: Quality costs. Quality costs are seen as a balance between failure costs and process improvement costs. The minimum quality cost occurs when failure costs and process improvement costs are equal.

ANALYZING THE BUSINESS AS A SYSTEM

Deming and Shewhart were physicists, and they brought applied statistics to the line level. TQM practitioners can go a long way without any statistical background or formal training in it. But at some point, to grasp the full import of these lessons, it is important for them to at least think like statisticians. Operations and processes must be viewed in a different light, one that does not use conventional cause-and-effect analysis. The key to applying TQM is the understanding of process variation.

In Figure 1.7 the laboratory is shown as the system with raw materials being converted into product. The inherent error of such a system is comprised of many diverse components. For example, a badly designed system will result in poor reporting reliability. It is important to recognize that the reliability of such a system can never rise above the latent error or design error inherent in the system and its component processes. Conversely, as the reliability of the component processes is improved, the overall system reliability improves according to well-known rules of probability.

Figure 1.8 shows a system which consists of an ordering department, a testing department, and a reporting department. Suppose that these all perform at an A average or with a 90 percent reliability. The probability of doing the right thing, or simply doing well, is 0.9. This is the reliability. The probability of the entire system working, that is, the correct order taken, the testing done right, and the report written and transmitted correctly, is $0.9 \times 0.9 \times 0.9 = 0.73$. In other words, the overall system works at a C average. Not very good.

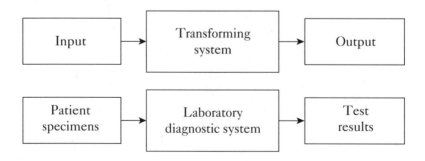

Figure 1.7: The laboratory as a diagnostic system. The lab may be thought of as a simple system in which specimens for analysis are received, tested, and reported.

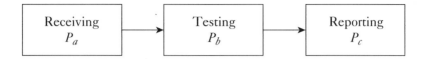

Figure 1.8: Three-part lab system. In this lab system, the overall reliability is the product of the individual reliabilities or P (overall) $= P_a \times P_b \times P_c$.

Now suppose that each step is reviewed in the department before it proceeds; that is, the ordering is reviewed and the testing and reporting have built-in quality checks. Assume that these quality check operations are no better than the operation themselves; that is, they are operating at 90 percent reliability also.

The improvement in each system is given by $R = 1 - (1 - P_a)(1 - P_b)$ $= 1 - (1 - 0.9)(1 - 0.9) = 1 - (0.1)(0.1) = 1 - 0.01 = 0.99$. Thus the overall reliability of the three-component system is $0.99 \times 0.99 \times 0.99 = 0.97$. Big difference. This shows the importance of review. This is built into lab work on several levels: the Food and Drug Administration (FDA) requires a second signature on process work, and Health Care Finance Administration (HCFA) requires that abnormals be repeated.

This is the reasoning behind this sort of requirement, the double check. It also shows that without the review process, various interacting departments, all performing at A average productivity, when combined into a larger system, can cause the larger system to fail. This is a case of A's not being good enough.

PROCESS IMPROVEMENT AND
THE TOOLS OF THE TQM TRADE

Process improvement, and hence improvement in the business, are aimed at eliminating or minimizing special variation in the process or system. Initially, a process is identified and is brought under control. A variable or attribute, which reflects the system performance, is used to monitor the process capability as it currently exists.

The improvement process, shown in Figure 1.9, identifies the difference between current performance and improved performance as a performance gap. This avoids describing the difference in negative terms such as problem solving. The techniques can be used for problem solving, but this

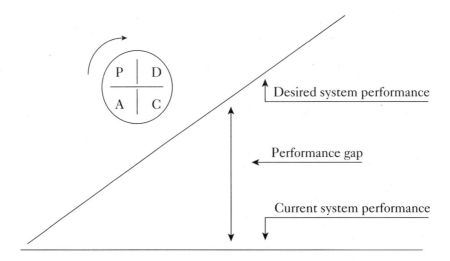

Figure 1.9: The performance gap. The performance gap is the observable difference between the current system performance and the desired system performance. Closing the gap is done by skillful application of the PDCA process.

perspective loses the viewpoint of system improvement and will tend to revert the technique back to a goal-oriented process. Instead, the idea is to reach the level of improved performance using the TQM tools in the fashion dictated by the PDCA cycle.

Achieving the process improvement is done by skilled application of various tools which have been developed to do this. Additionally, the Japanese have developed the seven new tools which are directed at predicting system shortcomings before they cause problems. In this sense, they are used in the planning phase of the Deming cycle. These seven new tools are

1. Affinity diagram
2. Interrelationship diagraph
3. Systematic diagram
4. Matrix diagram
5. Matrix data analysis
6. Process decision program chart (PDPC) analysis
7. Arrow diagrams

The quality control (QC) tools are used from the onset to analyze problems and to identify the paths to process improvement. These seven QC tools are

1. Flowchart
2. Ishikawa cause-and-effect (fishbone) diagram
3. Check sheet
4. Histogram and pareto diagram
5. Run chart/control chart
6. Scatter diagram
7. Stratification

These 14 tools and their uses are reviewed in detail in chapter 4. Further, there are four advanced tools which are (1) design of experiments, (2) Taguchi analysis, (3) multivariate analysis, and (4) regression analysis. These are discussed in chapters 4 and 6.

The most important step in making the process improvement stick is to ascribe ownership of the process, generally to supervision, line, or middle management, so that someone is continually responsible for maintaining the process at the new level. Juran, in *Managerial Breakthrough*, reviews the Japanese view reflecting his teachings to them. Basically, the Japanese recognize two main functions of the manager: to affect the quantum jump in process performance and to maintain the process at the new level of effectiveness. To accomplish this, the manager must understand the process, understand process variation, and accept ownership of the process and its improvement. This ownership and acceptance is guaranteed by a high-level audit function. Here, all ongoing processes are reviewed on an annual or semiannual basis by top management, which goes down to the floor to conduct interviews and reviews with the line personnel to assure the managers that the new processes are, in fact, being heeded and observed.

THE SIX-SIGMA GOAL

Motorola, the first winner of the Baldrige award, has popularized the term *six sigma*. The phrase relates to an error rate of only 3.4 per million. It comes from an off-center, normally distributed probability function capability index of $C_{pk} = 1.5$ with the standardized normal variable $z = 4.5$. Irrespective of the origin, the goal has become part of the quality literature. In effect, Motorola has said that all of its production error, which includes random error of 4.5 standard deviations, and constant error of 1.5 standard deviations, should be less than 3.4 mistakes in a million tries. This definition of process capability and capability ratio is more clearly shown in chapter 6, on statistics. In particular, see Figures 6.5 and 6.6.

From this, U.S. modern management gets six sigma as a performance goal. It wants to limit overall process variation to a unilateral tolerance of 3.4 errors in one million operations. A typical evaluation of this sort of operation appeared in *Business Month* (1990), "Stalking Six Sigma."[4]

The six-sigma goal concept can be traced to TQM via Shewhart and Juran, so the concept would appear to be a good one. In many instances this is the case; management identifies the six-sigma goal as a doable thing, and begins to provide the planning and support to reach the goal. In other cases, however, it can be an unrealistic zero-defect strategy which runs counter to Deming's instructions to focus on the process and let the goals be achieved inevitably by reduction in process variation.

This is a good example of another goal that Deming says to avoid. It is sometimes difficult to follow Deming and his anathematic attitude toward goal setting. It would sometimes appear as if quality goals are respectable. The idea is to get performance as good as possible, and it would seem that this is achieved by setting quality goals as rigorously as possible. Deming says absolutely not. Once again, he says, focus on the process and the variation in it. The quality goals will attain naturally.

If a watch runs five minutes fast every day, it will continue to do so until the error is adjusted out. No amount of training education, incentive, or criticism will make the watch give correct time.

This is a pivotal point. One of the problems in understanding it comes from the quality control charts just mentioned. These are rational goals based on instrument performance which are used in SPC. Limits of acceptability must be set for the process variation, and causes of unacceptable variation must be eliminated. Setting the acceptance limits for the process is addressing the allowable variation in the process. Who sets these limits? The customer does. Whatever limits are acceptable to the customer define the limit of variation allowable in the service setting. If a watch setting with a constant five-minute bias is acceptable to the wearer, then his or her quality goal has been met. If not, the wearer must take a management role and change the system performance.

It can be a mistake to set too rigorous limits, if the customer doesn't want them. It simply costs the company extra money in a tail-chasing effort to hit a quality goal that nobody but management wants. The key in setting these goals correctly is making absolutely certain the customer's voice has been heard correctly. Companies do not, for the most part, have sufficiently substantial programs to monitor the customer's voice. In fact, even with very good programs, the customer is not always easy to hear. With a substandard monitoring program it is almost guaranteed that what the customer gets is what the company wants to deliver, which can be what the customer is accepting but not necessarily wanting. If someone else offers the customer something nearer the desired mark, watch how fast that customer leaves.

Deming has noted, however, that "the customer never invented anything, not the light bulb, not the pneumatic tire." Deming's point is that the customer will generally define what he or she would like to see more or less of. Occasionally the customer will bring some item to a company which may be an interesting plus.

For instance, doctors hear of new test offerings in continuing educational conferences which they may pass on to the lab. The customer, however, will never create a technological breakthrough or innovation for the company. This must be generated internally, and the process and planning structure must accommodate this. If it does not, the company will continue to produce better technology of the status quo. This technology will gradually become obsolete.

Deming asks, "What happened to the carburetor manufacturers?" In 1987 a Honda Accord was manufactured in three models, a DX, an LX, and an LXi. Only the LXi had fuel injection, the other two had conventional carburetors. With the 1990 models, Honda was almost the last to go to completely fuel-injected cars. This happened fast. Deming's point is that breakthrough innovation is key to continued long-term productivity, and it won't be found by polling the customer. The customer's views need to be garnered in order to set acceptable limits to service quality, but they cannot be relied upon to keep the company abreast of competition.

Florida Power & Light

In the book *Deming Management at Work* Mary Walton recounts various TQM success stories of U.S. companies. It would appear, at first glance, that this is the missing link between Japanese TQC and American TQM—the proof that Japanese methods work on U.S. soil with U.S. workers, and hence, are not limited to Japanese shops. This is particularly true for FPL which was a nearly pure Japanese TQC effort.

In speaking with several FPL people from their former president Robert Tallon through middle managers and line workers, the conclusion is irresistible that TQC worked well there, but also had a fatal flaw. The key indicators for productivity all show quite conclusively that TQC worked as advertised. Complaints to the Public Service Commission went down, power generated per unit fuel input went up, equipment downtime was reduced, and power outages were minimized. Line workers loved it. Prior to TQC, maintenance people wouldn't answer their phones after 4:30 P.M. for fear of being called over to fix a steam leak or other equipment malfunction.

Middle management on the other hand, viewed TQC as a fine thing in many respects, but managers were driven nearly to distraction to collect data for the Japanese Deming Prize inspection committee. This went on to such an extent that one manager said to me, "They just forgot that we weren't Japanese." It appears that this disregard for the human element in a nearly fanatical bid for the prize ultimately cost upper management the staff support it needed and finally led the current FPL management group to abandon the system entirely.

It is not uncommon for a company to falter after receiving the Deming Prize. There can be a period of reassessment following the award. The FPL reaction was particularly acute due to a number of factors, only one of which—the missing human element—related to TQM.

It is still logical, however, that if TQM could work in Japan, given the country's prior reputation for poor manufacturing and its war-torn devastation, it can work in the United States, as well as or better than in any other country in present times. This is true with a single, very important caveat, and this is the embellishment added by Deming himself in his theory of profound knowledge. Deming management incorporates a humanistic element which was missing from Japanese TQC, an omission which some believe contributed to its ultimate failure at FPL, and may eventually result in its downfall or modification in Japan as well.

THE THEORY OF PROFOUND KNOWLEDGE

The theory of profound knowledge was first formulated by Deming at the Institute of Management Sciences conference in Osaka in 1989. The provisional status of the 14 points is entirely absent from the theory. Whereas many of the 14 points aren't applicable in Japan, the theory has universal appeal and applicability. Deming says that to properly apply TQM, a fundamental understanding of four major points must be undertaken. These are (1) a knowledge of system theory, (2) knowledge of the theory of variation, (3) an understanding of the theory of knowledge, that is, how people learn, and (4) an understanding of psychology, that is, why people do what they do.

Without an understanding of these points, Deming believes that applying TQM in one's own business based on the experience of others in other situations won't work. This theory is explored in detail in the next chapter.

NOTES

1. David Halberstam, *The Reckoning* (New York: Avon Books, 1986), p. 313.

2. Ibid., p. 315.

3. Philip B. Crosby, *Quality Is Free* (New York: McGraw Hill, 1979).

4. Mark Stuart Gill, "Stalking Six Sigma," *Business Month* (January 1990).

SUGGESTED READING

Abelson, Philip H. "The Lost U.S. Excellence in Manufacturing." *Science* 248 (April 13, 1990): 125

Deming, W. Edwards. *Out of the Crisis*. Cambridge, Mass.: MIT Center for Advanced Engineering Study, 1986.

Gitlow, Howard S., and Process Management International. *Planning for Quality, Productivity, and Competitive Position*. Homewood, Ill: Dow Jones-Irwin, 1990.

Ishikawa, Kaoru. *What Is Total Quality Control? The Japanese Way*. Englewood Cliffs, N. J.: Prentice-Hall, 1985.

Juran, J. M., and Frank M. Gryna. *Quality Planning and Analysis*. 3d ed. New York: McGraw-Hill, 1993.

Juran, J. M., ed. *Juran's Quality Control Handbook*. 4th ed. New York: McGraw-Hill, 1988.

Quality Digest (magazine). Red Bluff, Calif.: QCI International, March 1992.

Schroeder, Roger D. *Operations Management,* 3d ed. New York: McGraw-Hill, 1989.

Walton, Mary. *Deming Management at Work.* New York: G. P. Putnam's Sons, 1990.

2

Deming's Theory of Profound Knowledge

INTRODUCTION

Deming made a major addition to his management philosophy by formulating the theory of profound knowledge.[1] In some respects the subjects he proposed were unexpected. Many had anticipated that at this point, having recently given the world the 14 points, he would have built on this foundation and laid out a practical plan for implementing these points in a business setting. Instead, Deming said that to truly understand how to do business, it was more important to understand the foundation upon which the 14 points stand, and this he called profound knowledge.

Deming said that profound knowledge derives from four major areas of study. These are

- The theory of systems
- The theory of variation
- The theory of knowledge
- The understanding of psychology

Deming refers to a system as a series of functions or activities within an organization that work together for the aim of the organization. He views a

33

business as a system of interacting management processes, responsive to market needs, which can be analyzed and improved. Regarding the current business school offerings, Deming believes that a school of business ought to teach profound knowledge as a system. He says that "a school of business has the obligation to prepare students for the future, not the past. At present, most schools of business teach students how business is conducted, and how to perpetuate the present system of management—exactly what we don't need."[2]

THE THEORY OF SYSTEMS

From the remarks delivered at Osaka, Deming indicates that the following points represent the foundations of profound knowledge.

- Competition versus cooperation
- The Taguchi loss function
- Interdependency of systems
- Problem prioritization (Pareto analysis)
- Flowcharting

Competition Versus Cooperation

The 1980s was the decade of business acquisition and consolidation. Rather than supporting startups and new ventures, existing businesses were joined, and staffs were streamlined to eliminate redundancy.

Deming claims that the value of competition is misleading in the workplace, and that, instead, cooperation should be fostered. He adds that new markets should be sought rather than market segments increased, which acquisition and consolidation undeniably do.

One way to find new markets is to create them through innovation, and the Japanese are supporting research efforts in a big way. While America invests its money into bailing out the savings and loans, paying interest on the national debt, underwriting health care, and propping up tottering industries, Japan invests in R&D.

On an individual basis, the business culture and environment should foster a situation where people help each other to maximize their individual strengths. This will happen in a group that is rewarded for its output. In a group in which individual effort is rewarded (employee of the month, top salesperson, and so on), individual efforts and self-promotion are the rule. Individual recognition and promotion of individual efforts will also tend to maximize costs. In a system like that, sharing breakthrough technology or systems would be self-defeating. From the company's perspective, it is best that all employees function at maximum capability. To achieve this, some employees are going to have to sacrifice their own self-interests to promote the welfare and growth of others. If this is not recognized and supported by the company, then it is unlikely to be done except by the most altruistic individuals, and altruism is a humanitarian virtue little valued in most business climates.[3]

The Taguchi Loss Function and Interdependency of Systems

The Taguchi loss function is a quadratic expression which describes the loss to society as a process delivery moves away from the nominal delivery. Figure 2.1 shows the Taguchi perspective as opposed to zero-defect thinking. The concept of the difference is important and not well understood. Zero-defects thinking is goalpost thinking. Anything that meets specifications is okay. This leads to viewing process components as little islands of individual activity without regard for their interaction with other steps in the process.

The Taguchi philosophy focuses on the interaction of systems. Deming recognizes that each system will have an input and an output and that the output of one system can be used as the input for another. If this is the case, then it is important that these systems function in harmony.

The example in Figure 2.2 of a large bolt going into a small nut may seem trivial, but think about it next time you are using a snap-top aspirin

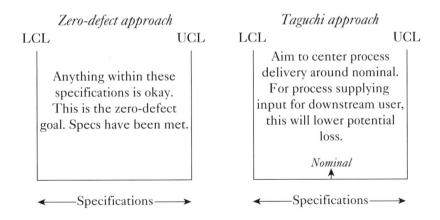

Figure 2.1: Taguchi loss function. Between the upper and lower control limits (UCL/LCL) the treatment of variation between these two methods is quite different.

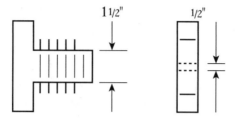

Figure 2.2: Zero defects and specification limits. This is a one-and-one-half-inch bolt trying to go into a half-inch nut. The specifications for each were one inch, plus or minus a half inch. From a zero-defects perspective, both parts meet specifications.

bottle. Then think also of the flowchart of a process as being important so that the individual steps are not simply sequential, but must be integrated so as to function in harmony. This requires that process delivery be centered as closely as possible around the nominal delivery reference point.

In the lab, for instance, if the technical and reporting functions are separate, then technical data can't simply be dumped into reporting. The two systems must interact smoothly to effect a timely and accurate transfer of the technical work onto the final report and finally to the end user.

Pareto Analysis and Flowcharting

Deming's reference to the tools of Japanese TQC is an indication that he views these as an important part of his management style as well. These are discussed at some length in later chapters and it does not pay to belabor the obvious. It is important, however, that they were referenced in the profound knowledge statements, because reading Deming's 14 points leaves one somewhat unclear as to where he stands with regard to the more practical aspects of TQM implementation and deployment.

THE THEORY OF VARIATION

The following points which Deming views as important for managers to know can be extracted from his theory.

- Normal variation
- Stable and unstable processes
- Process capability
- Special- and common-cause variation

- Tampering, chaos theory, and funnel experiments
- Statistical theory of failure (reliability)
- Statistical process control
- Sampling theory

Remember it is important to think like a statistician. The points Deming raises can be discussed from a theoretical standpoint without ever using a chart, graph, or equation. This is one of the wonderful things about TQM, that it is possible, without a doctorate in statistics, to integrate these views into all levels of the workplace and into the quality of daily work.

Bringing statistics to the line is one of Deming's major contributions, and Deming's focus on this area brings into view how statistics fits into the overall picture. Statistics in the lab consist mainly of quality control charts. Deming's message is that a fuller understanding of the philosophy of statistical thought should pervade all thinking about process control, performance, improvement, and delivery.

Normal Variation, Stable and Unstable Processes, Process Capability, and Special- and Common-Cause Variation

These subjects are reviewed in considerable detail in chapter 6. A capsule view here, however, may help give additional perspective.

A process that is in statistical control will have an output which varies about a mean value ($\overline{X}$). The variation (R) can be expressed in terms of standard deviation (s.d.), or percent coefficient of variation (% CV). Lab managers frequently find themselves in the position of reacting to statements such as, "The number of unbilled ER charge tickets is way up" and "Many clients aren't getting their reports on time."

To respond to these statements, management must conduct a statistical review of the process in question. Most of the time it will be found that when the mean and two s.d. of the process delivery are plotted, that the "way-up" excursion is within the statistical process capability. In other words, the process is continuing to deliver what it has always delivered, and from the critical remarks received, this may not be good enough.

To correct the excursion is to improve process delivery. This can be done by first ensuring that the process is stable; that is, that it continues to deliver the same output with time. That the process hasn't any special-cause variability must also be determined. This is the variability that is under operator control and can be fixed by working with the operator. Common cause is the error associated with management control and is insensitive to operator critique or incentive systems. In either case, the data must be examined and plotted, and the system must be analyzed for plausibility and possibly critiqued by the use of failure mode and effect analysis and fault tree analysis (see chapter 4). As the experts say, "Let the data talk to you."

Tampering, Chaos Theory, and Funnel Experiments

A powerful example of overreaction to normal process variation is the funnel experiment. The purpose of the funnel experiment is to show how overcontrol or tampering results in a system eventually oscillating out of control and exhibiting chaotic behavior.

A funnel is firmly suspended above a sheet of paper and a steel pellet allowed to repeatedly fall through the funnel onto the paper. Each time the pellet falls through, the spot where the pellet hits the paper is marked by a dot. After enough repetitions the resulting pattern looks like Figure 2.3, sort of like a fuzzy donut.

This turns out to be the system delivery; that is, the best precision and accuracy the system can muster. The only way to improve on this is through a system change which would be to make the funnel hole smaller or to move the funnel closer to the paper.

As an example of tampering, it is possible to "correct" the funnel position each time the pellet falls through. This can be done using graph

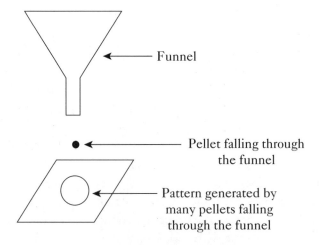

Figure 2.3: The funnel experiment. This is the pattern generated by pellets falling through the funnel which remains stationary.

paper and compensating the funnel position as a result of where the pellet lands; in essence, if it lands too far left, move the funnel to the right an equal amount. Deming actually uses three different corrective measures, each of which results in a pattern wider than the donut, and two actually become chaotic and blow up.

At one time chaos theory was considered a theory in search of an application, because the equations associated with this area of research are nonlinear and can't be solved except by brute force; that is, trying solutions and seeing if they fit the equation. With computers, they can now do the same thing, but it doesn't take the lifetime of a dedicated scientist to come up with a single solution. As a result, more applications of chaos theory are coming into use in all phases of inquiry.

The butterfly effect is often used as an example of chaotic behavior. Systems that can be described by these methods are extremely sensitive to initial conditions. Additionally, the output is unpredictable from initial conditions, but is describable (once it occurs) by various fractal sets. The butterfly effect is an example derived from weather forecasting, because this was one of the first efforts to use fractals, and refers to the flapping of a butterfly's wings miles away, eventually causing a sandstorm over the Sahara Desert. In chapter 3 one aspect of chaos in the Cantor Dust is mentioned. Here, it is shown how redundancy or foolproofing is one way of improving the reliability of a process. Deming refers to chaos not only in this instance, but also in the field of sampling theory, which will be explored in more detail later.

The Figure 2.3 shows an example of the funnel experiment while the funnel remains stationary. Figure 2.4 shows one of the chaotic, tampered patterns, sometimes called the running-man or bow-tie pattern.

The funnel experiment is a lesson for managers who are continually twiddling with a process to see if minor corrective adjustments and counternudges can result in improved system performance. This is frequently the attribute of managers who are after quick results and try to achieve this by hiring, firing, or shifting people around within a system in hopes of seeing improvement. Deming tries to show that the outcome of this tampering will be limited by the system delivery capabilities, and that tampering is likely to produce just the opposite effect from the one the managers want.

Other examples of tampering are whimsically changing the company insurance or retirement plan, and changing suppliers or vendors to see if

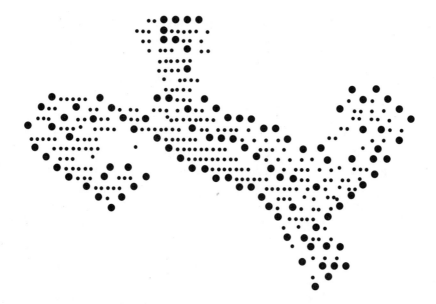

Figure 2.4: A funnel pattern with tampering. This is the figure generated by correcting the funnel position after each pellet drop.

another one can do better than the current one. The outset is that eventually there is no driving impetus behind the relationship except the dollar, and the dollar doesn't incorporate quality concerns.

Automatic process control, or operator adjustment of the instrument when the adjustment is within the process capabilities, will frequently result is sawtooth control charts. If the process is operating within the process capability limits, no adjustment can be made that will improve the process delivery. If the machine is out of control, then the special cause is corrected. If the adjustment is necessary due to wear or other problems not readily correctable, then the adjustment is made relative to a standard.

Gitlow et al. add the following examples of tampering. Using the last piece of the log sawed off to measure the next piece may sound trite, but consider the following:[4]

1. Making up a production shortage from the last period in the next period, or setting a current sales goal based on the shortfall from the last sales goal.

2. Cascading by having trainers teach others who then train still others. The process must be standardized with videos, check sheets, and standard manuals.

3. Setting policy based on the last set of data. Policy setting must be done with in-depth review of the component processes and with a thorough, long-term understanding of what is going on.

4. Evaluating people based on hearsay. This is also an example of tampering where the last rumor is used to initiate new policy regarding an individual or group. This will lead to personal self-aggrandizement of individuals and little group effort. If the rumor mill is the only way information reaches the supervisors, then it is in the individual's best interests to be as personally visible as possible, and to glorify oneself and belittle others. Cooperation and working to better the group or department are suppressed.

5. Changing company policy by using the latest employee survey as a criterion for change. Taking the pulse of employee attitudes is important in understanding the general attitude and outlook of the staff. Certainly the company should be responsive in all areas that will engender a workplace in keeping with employee satisfaction and inspiration. Policy, though, is generated in keeping with the company's mission statement. That statement is integrated into customer requirements in keeping with stated company values and beliefs.

Statistical Theory of Failure (Reliability), Statistical Process Control, and Sampling Theory

These are three areas of statistics which are not easily explained in any depth without some formulas and some examples of applications. The concepts can be explained, however, without much math, and the concepts are important to use when planning and implementing TQM. As long as these ideas are appreciated, then the statistical resource group can supply the methods to effect measurement and analysis plans. In the next section, the concept of reliability is discussed, and in the chapter on statistics, the details of sampling theory and statistical process control are reviewed.

Reliability

Figure 2.5 shows the failure rate over time of a complex piece of equipment. This has been called the bathtub curve. The curve can be thought of as having three distinct areas. The first is the infant mortality region. In this time period, unanticipated early failure takes place. It is very costly to manufacturers, as the equipment is generally warranted during this period. Much design thought goes into reducing these early failures. One method of keeping these units out of consumers' hands is burn-in. This is when each unit is stress tested prior to shipment.

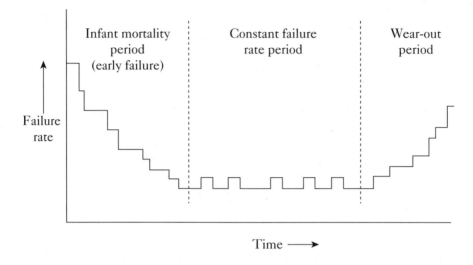

Figure 2.5: A failure or bathtub curve. This is a curve which qualitatively expresses the three regions into which the failure of complex equipment may be categorized. The first area is the infant mortality period during which failure occurs soon after production. This is sometimes forestalled by manufacturers during a burn-in period in which the equipment is run under conditions of stress prior to sale. The second area is described by zero-order kinetics, a constant failure rate, and, if characterized well enough, allows manufacturers to create warranty and service contracts that reflect this. The third area is the one reflecting senescence and frequent repair of the equipment. This is generally an out-of-warranty time period that is expensive for the customer and indicates that replacement is the best course.

The second area of the curve is the region of constant failure rate. This region allows some statistical calculations to be done using an exponential function to represent the kinetics. From these expressions, values can be derived such as mean time between failures (MTBF), and availability. Availability, or the fraction of time the instrument is up and running, versus being out of service, is an important number to know in scheduling and costing.

The third region of the bathtub curve is the time period in which the instrument becomes senescent and needs frequent repair. It should be replaced prior to repair cost escalation.

Figure 2.6 shows an analogous diagram of process (rather than instrument) decay which Imai portrays as happening without the reinforcement of

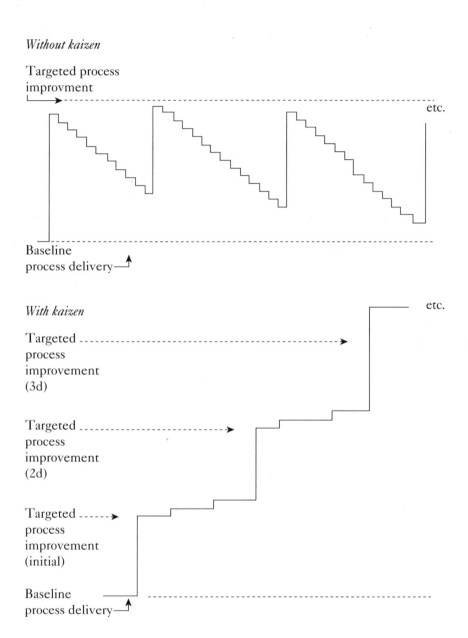

Figure 2.6: Process performance with time, with and without continuous improvement.

kaizen, or continuous process improvement.[5] Other authors refer to an entropic disintegration of a process if constant vigilance by the process owner and process improvement by the appropriate quality group does not ensue.

The second panel in Figure 2.6 shows the effect of kaizen on the process. The gradual unraveling of the process due to unauthorized deviation from policy is not only counteracted, but the process also is gradually improved in small ways prior to the next turn of the PDCA wheel. This results in a major step toward function improvement.

Metrics and Key Indicators

In closing this section, a brief discussion of the concepts of metrics and key indicators is appropriate. These terms arise from time to time in discussions of TQM efforts.

A metric is a variable chosen for measurement which represents an item in a component process. For instance, an automobile transmission may have a main bearing which must be manufactured to close tolerance or wear will result. The metric may be a principal bearing dimension such as the internal radius.

Key indicators (KIs) are used by companies to plot major system delivery which reflects company progress in a given area. For example, the number of transmission failures with time could be a key indicator of which the variation in bearing diameter would be just one metric which contributed to KI performance.

THE THEORY OF KNOWLEDGE

Deming begins by saying that any rational plan, however simple, requires prediction about conditions and behavior and comparison of performance of different procedures or materials. Thus if processes are going to be improved, then the two processes—the existing process and the improved process—must be compared. One must see if the difference results in improvement, and if the improvement justifies the means.

Deming believes that the job of top management is one of prediction. Data gathering and evaluation have to be accompanied by a testable theory and experimental design to enable the right predictions to be made with a high degree of confidence.

Currently management relies on experience, gut feel, and intuition to reach the conclusions upon which it bases decisions. Deming says that experience is no help to management unless it is studied with the aid of theory. To copy an example of success, without using theory to understand it, may lead to disaster.

Deming would probably be happy to add that the application of TQM without an understanding of the theory of profound knowledge is also an invitation to disaster. Quite a bit of TQM application in western society is passed off as "quality is everybody's job" with little additional substantive theory or application. Deming is making a case for a deeper understanding of theory and application.

Deming goes on to say that no particular number of examples establishes a theory, but that a single unexplained failure of a theory requires modification or even abandonment of it. This is a good argument for a thorough understanding of the seven management tools and the advanced tools, such as design of experiments, and the use of outcomes from these processes in system change and improvement.

Finally, Deming says that an empirical observation is subject to the observer's perspective. Any two people may have different ideas about what is important to know about any event. This is a profound truth. In a practical sense it leads to rigorous assignment of study variables and an enhanced respect for the group assignment of priorities via the affinity diagram and Pareto analysis.

THE UNDERSTANDING OF PSYCHOLOGY

In the discussion of psychology Deming focuses on several issues. He addresses the need for a deeper understanding of the principal element of the work force, the people who make it up. He makes the following points.

1. Understand people and their interaction with the business system. The understanding must be of a fundamental nature, and it must address reasons for people's behavior and interaction both with their peers and with members of different hierarchical groups.
2. Acknowledge that people are individuals and are different. Business currently operates as if all workers are the same.
3. Make allowances and install programs which recognize that people learn in different ways and at different speeds.

4. Organize a company to run based on intrinsic rather than extrinsic motivation. Emphasize participation aimed at minimizing the Taguchi loss function for a process rather than conformance to specifications, which is essentially zero-defect thinking.

The Psychology and Physiology of Behavior

This is a field in which TQM offers the most opportunity for improvement and new insights. Since Deming was a mathematical physicist, and Juran was trained as an engineer and as an attorney, people concerns and understanding of these were not an initial focus of TQC as it was deployed in Japan and later, in perhaps its most spectacular western example, at FPL.

This partially reflects the progress of psychology and its contributions over the years to the understanding of human thought and behavior. For years it was thought that human beings were born into this world with a brain which was a tabula rasa, a blank slate, upon which their cumulative experiences were subsequently written. This created adult humans with all their prejudices, fears, hopes, creativity, and ambitions. The belief that all human behavior was learned was espoused by the behaviorist school of thought led by such people as B. F. Skinner and his colleagues.

Following the understanding of the double helix and the beginning of molecular biology, which offered new insights into how DNA passes on physical characteristics from generation to generation, new schools of behavior began to arise based on the assumption that if physical attributes could be inherited, perhaps behavior could also. Paul MacLean was first to point out that the brain could be thought of as having three distinct anatomical sections which related to the reptilian, mammalian, and human aspects of the evolutionary past.[6] These sections are both physically distinct, and, MacLean believed, intellectually dissimilar. The underlying message of MacLean is that humans have brought evolutionary baggage with them from their remote past and that it influences their behavior.

Examples are the fight or flight reflex frequently manifested as an irrational fear of public speaking and a fear of flying. Fear of flying may come from times in which the remote ancestors were arboreal, and falling down from trees was really dangerous. Speaking in front of a large group totally exposes the individual physically, emotionally, and intellectually. Neither of these fears is particularly amenable to counseling or reason. They seem to come without warning and depart just as mysteriously. MacLean and his group hypothesize that these fears do not reside with the higher brain functions, the ones which make humans rational and reason-able human beings, but deeper down where more primitive intellectual forces reside. At one time these sensitivities were very important for sur-vival in the trees or on the open savannah where humans with no long teeth or claws were at a severe physical disadvantage.

Roger W. Sperry of California Institute of Technology has spent the last 25 years producing a considerable body of knowledge about brain func-tion which is being carried on by his students, colleagues, and supporters around the world.[7] Sperry won the 1981 Noble Prize in medicine and physi-ology for this work.

The brain is divided into two hemispheres which are joined by a spaghetti-sized connection called the corpus callosum. Initially Sperry worked with animals and later with people who had suffered damage from stroke or trauma to a single side of the brain. His study results portray the brain as composed of two hemispheres which operate somewhat indepen-dently and have areas of specialization. In particular, the left brain having both Broca's and Wernicke's area, specializes in speech. If this area is dam-aged the person is left with different kinds of speech problems.

The right side of the brain appears to be related to more holistic and spatial insights such as artistic and creative distinctions. For instance, a per-son who is aphasic (can't speak) due to left hemisphere damage may still be able to sing songs with words perfectly well.

Since Sperry's research, psychologists and anthropologists elected to do far-reaching studies on identical twins. It had been noted anecdotally that twins not only look alike but they also seem to think and act alike. It was still argued by the behaviorists, however, that this was an environmen-tal imprinting, and that if genetics had anything to do with behavior, twin studies didn't prove anything. Then the Minnesota Study of Twins Reared Apart was published in 1991, followed by other studies which reported on identical twins who were reared in entirely different environments, with no knowledge of their sibling's whereabouts or circumstances. In these remarkable studies, the researchers found strong correlation in the personal behavior of the twins with regard to religion, sexual proclivity, job choice, number of children, hobbies, and general deportment which went far beyond happenstance.

For years, American business has been run as if people were infinitely malleable and that anyone could do anything and enjoy it as long as supervi-sion was thorough enough in its training and determined enough to make workers do the right thing. An analysis of these studies, however, indicates that people are not fully amenable to all situations, and that a job preference may be a reflection both of learning and genetic makeup.

In 1954 A. H. Maslow said that human needs could be thought of as forming a sort of hierarchy in which more basic needs, once satisfied, would be replaced by more esoteric needs. He believed that physiological needs relating to subsistence formed the base of the hierarchy and that, if satisfied, the individual would tend to focus on needs related to security. Further up the hierarchy would be social needs relating to group acceptance, ego satisfaction such as respect for self and by others, and finally self-fulfillment resulting in creativity and various forms of expression (see Table 2.1).

Maslow's hierarchy of human needs was popularized by Douglas McGregor, who recognized for the first time, the human side of productivity. This is in contrast to the earlier work of Frederick W. Taylor, who proposed separating the planning functions from execution. Taylor's theory, later called the theory of scientific management, was structured in this way from the belief that workers were not well educated and hence incapable of helping in the planning segment of management.

Although times have changed to the extent that many workers, particularly licensed laboratory workers, are more skilled in their jobs than the general administration that guides overall policy, the Taylor theory has become entrenched in western management, and line people rarely

Table 2.1: Maslow's hierarchy of human needs.*

Need	*Motivator*
1. *Physiological:* Basic survival, shelter, food. Need for subsistence income.	1. Bonuses, other cash rewards for good work.
2. *Security:* Need to continue at or above subsistence level.	2. Good work is rewarded by job security. No capricious layoffs.
3. *Social:* Group acceptance.	3. Team play emphasis.
4. *Ego:* Self-respect and other-respect.	4. Pride of workmanship, nonfinancial rewards.
5. *Self-fulfillment:* Creativity and expression.	5. Chance to participate in planning and change.

*Source: A. H. Maslow, *Motivation and Personality* (New York: Harper Bros., 1954).

participate in planning decisions. Consequently, management makes decisions in a vacuum and frequently may deploy administrative edicts which are very difficult to live with on the line level.

More than one industrial psychologist has stated that once Maslow's hierarchy of needs are satisfied, workers are almost immune to general motivation or censuring. The point is that people work for different reasons other than industry fiscal goals. This school of thought believes that people must be fit to job positions that most suit them and that no amount of encouragement or castigation will get a right foot in a left shoe with time. This is in keeping with the Japanese view in which workers are put into positions they want, but more importantly, are put into groups in which they are judged to be compatible from a behavioristic standpoint.

In adopting Japanese views on behavior, it is interesting to note that the work of Sperry has been continued in Japan and has uncovered some interesting differences in the cerebral hemispheric activities of the native Japanese versus their western counterparts. These studies were done with radio-labeled sugars which allow geographical areas of the brain to be mapped as determined by localized energy requirements during different activities.

Sperry showed that while right-handed westerners were reading, the left hemisphere is dominant. The Japanese, however, have two written languages, Kanji and Kana. Figure 2.7 shows that Kanji is an older pictorial language in which the pictograph actually stands for something the word represents. Kana, on the other hand, is more like English in that the pictographs stand for abstract sounds.

The Japanese process Kana just like Americans process their written language—on the left side of the brain. Kanji, on the other hand, is processed on the right, similar to other people's brain activity when looking at a picture or hearing a song. This difference may account for the Japanese preference for business tools that are primarily pictorial in nature because they are more readily able to process and convert these into speech and action. This is speculation at this point, but it indicates that, in fact, humans are different and that these differences may extend into ways in which people interact and do business.

Parenthetically it may be noted that these unconscious behavior traits are not inherited but learned. This is demonstrated by Japanese who are reared in the West but who learn both languages by processing on the left side of the brain, just like westerners.

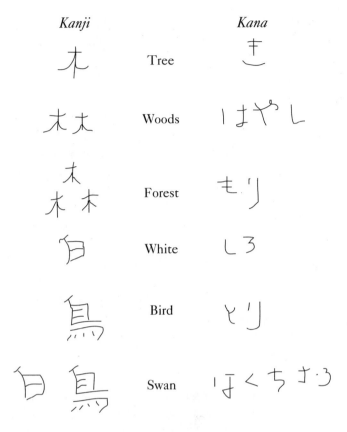

Figure 2.7: Kanji and Kana. Kanji uses symbols that are more pictorial than Kana. Kana uses symbols which stand for syllables. Japanese with damage to the left brain hemisphere lose the ability to read Kana, but can still read Kanji, since the visual-spatial activity resident in the right hemisphere is intact. This ability to process written concepts in either hemisphere may account for the Japanese predisposition to the seven quality and management tools, most of which reduce complex written or tabular data for pictorial presentation. *Source:* Bloom, Floyd. E. and Arlene Lazerson. *Brain, Mind and Behavior.* New York: W. H. Freeman, 1988.

East and West

It is very important to develop an understanding of the Japanese mentality, because in adapting TQC to the West some things work and others won't, based largely on cultural biases. Imai, in his book *Kaizen*, speaks of the Japanese process-oriented mentality in this way: "Japan's national sport is sumo. At each sumo tournament there are three awards: an outstanding performance award, a skill award, and a fighting spirit award. None of these three awards is based solely on results. This is a good example of Japan's process-oriented thinking."

Later Imai speaks of praying at a particular Shinto shrine.

A worshiper wishing to pray at the shrine altar has to walk through a dense forest, up steep stone steps, and through some 15,000 gates along the walkway. By the time the worshipper reaches the altar he is steeped in the sacred atmosphere. Getting there is almost as important as the prayer itself.

In the United States, no matter how hard a person works, lack of results will result in a poor personal rating and lower income or status. The individual's contribution is valued only for its concrete results. Only the results count in a result-oriented society.

Another often-misunderstood Japanese business adjunct is the quality circle. In the 1980s, American business got the idea that quality circles were the way to bring Japanese quality issues to the workplace and that doing so would automatically bring business the rewards that the Japanese were reaping. This was further fostered in a public television show, "If Japan Can, Why Can't We?" Of this show, Juran says, "I think that it has set this country back a decade by offering a completely oversimplified and misleading version of Japan's quality revolution."

Of the quality circles started in the early 1980s, it is estimated that only about one in eight still survive. This may change as TQM goes into the U.S. workplace, but whether the term quality circle will be much used in the United States is doubtful due to the dismal reputation for success it met here.

A more likely group becoming popular now is the process improvement group (PIG, task team, or quality action team). It is more like a SWAT team established to diagnose and implement process improvement. When the improvement is locked in, the maintenance is turned over to the proper ownership group and the PIG is dissolved.

Quality circles, on the other hand, are permanent fixtures, and are formed voluntarily. In Japan, 35 percent to 50 percent of workers are in one, and the circles have a national registry. Prizes are given to top-performing groups. As Imai says, "Most Japanese companies active in kaizen programs have a quality control system and a suggestion system working in concert. The role of the QC circles may be better understood if we regard them collectively as a group-oriented suggestion system."

The suggestion system is one of the key operational schemes in TQC. It is both a way of identifying opportunities from the workers' perspective and a way of voluntarily bringing workers into the improvement process.

Robert Tallon, the president of FPL during its quality revolution, said that at the peak of its progress FPL was getting about two to three suggestions per employee per year, or about 30,000 suggestions annually. Of those, management was able to respond to 75 percent within three to six months. Much higher suggestion rates are quoted for many Japanese companies. Imai says that one Japanese employee turned in over 15,000 individual suggestions in one year.

A change is required in U.S. industry. A suggestion system must be established that is responsive and works to keep submitters involved by letting them know that their counsel is worthy and that their input is being used. This can be done by a system in which the individuals are encouraged to work with the process improvement groups.

Other authors have pointed out that the Japanese culture encourages group activity and cooperation from birth. Young children are active in many community, social, and religious activities which are designed to instill in them the attitude that they are an integral part of a community process, and that even as they are dependent on it, it is also dependent on them.

This type of early Japanese training, which continues on through adolescence and into adulthood, is largely missing in the United States. In some of the more disadvantaged neighborhoods the teaching is diametrically opposed to the local ethic. Residents in these areas frequently feel polarized and only deal with the community on an adversarial basis. There, the attitude may be more how to survive and do well despite the system. This disparity is essential to understanding the deployment of some of the Japanese activities into the U.S. workplace and adapting them for use here.

Individuals responsible for the plantwide deployment of TQM are going to have to look closely at their own corporate culture and determine how, where, and to what extent to employ the many group activities which are so central to Japanese TQC. Careful thought must go into reward and incentive programs so that groups receive the rewards and recognition, and not, as so often is the case now, the individual.

Eastern and Western Businesspeople

In January 1992 President Bush sent a cadre of U.S. industrialists to Japan to soften the way prior to his own Asian tour. The leader of the group was Lee Iacocca, president of Chrysler Motors. This was deemed appropriate as Japan has a goodly share of the U.S. car market, a share that is growing larger each year. The senator from Michigan, Fortney "Pete" Stark, summed it all up by saying, "The current U.S. recession is the fault of Japan."

Now 1992 was an election year, and even though Americans are pretty immune to a politician's preelection rhetoric, such statements by elected representatives did little to cement lasting relations between the two countries. Stark's implication that Japan should make cars as inferior to those in the United States in order to balance the trade deficit overlooks the fact that, for years, U.S. industry manufactured and sold cars of poor quality all over the world where they fell apart just as quickly as here. If these other countries ever complained of the United States contributing to their trade deficit, it received little press here at the time, and even less interest by Congress.

In 1989 Shintiro Ishihara, an outspoken Japanese statesman, and Akio Morita, the chair of Sony Corporation, published a book titled *The Japan That Can Say No*. When a bootleg translation was circulated in this country, it caused such an uproar that Morita declined to be associated with the authorized English translation. It was published in 1991 and contains the following observation by Ishihara.[8]

> Mesmerized by junk bonds and leveraged buyouts, top U.S. management has contributed to the decline in American competitiveness. Profligate indebtedness has replaced frugality. Many executives seem uninterested in making profits the old-fashioned way: earning them with reliable products at affordable prices. Lee Iacocca, to cite one, was considered U.S. presidential timber, but by Japanese standards he is an unethical manager. In a cynical betrayal of American motorists, he took advantage of the appreciated yen that made imported Japanese cars more expensive, and jacked up the price of Chrysler cars. Iacocca also received huge bonuses after Chrysler employees had agreed to give backs to save the company.
>
> The United States may deplore Japan's status as the world's creditor, but it happened because the Reagan administration's plans backfired. In 1985 U.S. leaders were laughing up their sleeve at the dollar depreciation scheme they had foisted on Tokyo. It misfired and made Japan affluent. Americans should follow the Chinese proverb, "When things go wrong, first look in the mirror."

Men and Women

Sperry's hemispheric brain studies were originally done on soldiers whose brain trauma had been caused by injuries sustained in combat. Because these studies were all done on men, the original conclusions were biased in the same sense that the conclusions drawn in the cholesterol studies were biased by working with largely male populations.

It was found later, as more women were included in controlled studies, that women may have much higher cholesterol levels and not be in the same risk category as men. Similarly, the brain studies showed that whereas in men, the delegation of activities between the hemispheres is quite acute, in women there seems to be a more holistic way of handling vocal and analytical processes. This is particularly evident during recovery from stroke in which the female brain seems better able to transfer speech activities to the undamaged side, rather than lose them entirely which is frequently the case with males.

In a sense, this makes women as different from men in their analytical processes as Japanese are from westerners. Women exhibit this very young as they vocalize right brain functions such as showing the tender and sympathetic quality of playing with dolls, but, at the same time, continually talking about the process, a property which boys actually find rather baffling. This may continue as girls mature and learn about love and heterosexual bonding but reflect on it by spending hours talking over the details.

Dr. Deborah Tannen, author of *You Just Don't Understand*, is a linguist who suggests that these inherent differences in neural data processing may frequently result in communication obstacles between the sexes. This is just like the cultural differences which result in communications problems between the East and West even when both speak the same language. Tannen says,[9]

> Complementary Schismogenesis commonly sets in when men and women have divergent sensitivities and hypersensitivities. For example, a man who fears losing freedom will pull away at the first sign he views as an effort to control him, but pulling away is just the signal that sets off alarms for the woman who fears losing intimacy. Her attempts to get closer will aggravate his fear, and his reaction—pulling further away—will aggravate her in an ever-widening spiral. Understanding each other's styles, and the motives behind them, is a first step in breaking this destructive circuit.

Tannen goes on to show how many men prefer to use speech for communication whereas women may use it for this, as well as social interaction. She expresses concern about categorizing gender-specific communication since it tends to foster reductionist thinking that stereotypes the sexes with regard to their spoken communication. She is quick to point out that both sexes have valid perspectives and that understanding them is the key. She is also aware that "the male is seen as normative, the female as departing from the norm. And it is only a short step—maybe an inevitable one—from different to worse."

Nevertheless she observes, "Pretending that men and women are the same hurts women, because the ways they are treated are based on the norms for men. It also hurts men who, with good intentions, speak to women as they would to men, and are nonplussed when their words don't work as expected, or even spark resentment or anger."

Tannen has given many presentations on communication differences between various populations, not unlike the topics in this section of this book. Ninety percent of inquiries, however, centered around gender-specific topics that resulted in her book on this subject. It is clear that it is a subject that people want to know about, and it is particularly important in the business setting as industries shift from traditionally male-dominated management structures to a more equitable distribution of responsibilities.

The Role of Women in Japanese TQC

Dr. Howard Gitlow recently reflected on a trip he took to Japan with his wife Shelly. They both went as consultants to a major Japanese manufacturing firm. Shelly Gitlow is a specialist in the human relationships and human resources aspect of management. The meeting convened in an elegant, top-floor conference room. At one point Shelly asked where the ladies' room was. At the conference table were the top managers in the company, men who had been with the firm for many years. None of them knew where the women's restroom was located. They were uncertain if one even existed. Finally, in an epiphanic moment, one of the executives thought to find one of the women who serve refreshments during these meetings, a tea maid. This woman took Shelly on a winding, convoluted journey into the remote parts of the building until they finally located a women's restroom about a city block away from the main conference room.

The entire Japanese TQC effort was done entirely without female representation either in the work force or in the government. Japanese women had, however, a very important role in the maintenance of a stable family situation during the quality revolution. They saw to it that the children were thoroughly integrated into the Japanese culture and ethic and that they got all possible opportunities for education and training. Since the Japanese TQC effort has been underway for the past 45 years, this contribution has been critical. The women provided the community with the stabilizing support of the home environment in the very competitive business and educational world of Japan.

Dr. Marvin Harris, America's leading anthropologist authored *Our Kind, The Evolution of Human Life and Culture*. In it he reviews the evolutionary and developmental steps taken by humans on their path to modern society. He says,

> Large numbers of married mothers began to enter the wage labor forces in the 1960s with the intention of supplementing the family income. Thirty years later, the expansion and feminization of the labor force had driven the wage rates down, making a second income mandatory to pay for decent housing while decent children became an unaffordable luxury. How were these things decided?

In the March 13, 1992 issue of *Science*, there is a section called "Women in Science" which compares women in the job corps around the world. In Japan, women account for only 3 percent of all undergraduate and postgraduate students. There are no female professors or assistant professors of science or engineering. To redress this imbalance there are several advertisements for U.S. women scientists to come and work in Japan.

Old and Young

As Sperry's work encompassed a broad patient base, one of the conclusions drawn was the ability of older brains to show greater integration between the halves than younger brains. Older brains responded to damage and repair more like the female brain in this respect. One feature of older people is the potential for encompassing differences which, earlier in life, keep people apart.

In the East, Confucianism is a form of ancestor worship. One aspect of that culture, very different from the West, is the accommodation made for elderly workers. In this country, people get raises every year until they are overpaid for the functions they perform just by virtue of the fact that they have been doing their jobs for so long. This encourages managers to meet cost-savings goals by replacing older workers with younger and cheaper ones. In addition to saving some salary money, the company doesn't have to ultimately pay a retirement pension, and health care costs are less with a younger, insurable worker population.

In Japan, the wage scale is based on longevity also, but is scheduled to peak during the workers' years of maximum need. This is generally when the kids are in college. After this, the salary declines and as a result the workers don't find themselves cashiered because their salary has outstripped their contributions. In addition to this, the Japanese have an alternative career path for older workers in the areas of training and teaching younger workers and sharing with them the elders' knowledge and experience.

This fits with Drucker's remarks about the future strategy of Japanese industry. The Japanese feel that with all the investment they have in their skilled work force, mass production is something best done somewhere else. They speak instead of brain capital. Each company is establishing a research institute and its purpose, according to Drucker, is to "bring to the group awareness of any important new knowledge—in technology, in management and organization, in marketing, in finance, in training—developed worldwide."

On Learning

Teaching in this country has been standardized over the years. Generally it consists of a lecturer who presents a series of facts, at a measured rate, to an audience which takes notes. Later, students are given time to digest the presentation and to read more on the subject and perhaps work some problems in the subject.

Recently, it has been recognized that all people may not learn as well from a presentation as from other methods. It is now widely acknowledged that people learn differently—some alone, others in groups—some by reading, others by doing, and still others from hearing it described or perhaps by seeing it done.

Efforts now are being made to encompass these varied approaches and to individualize teaching methods. This way all people can be reached to the extent that they are able to learn the material, internalize it, and express it in their own particular way.

Throughout this process, every effort is made to standardize the course content so that everyone gets the same material. Course evaluations reflect that, in fact, everyone got the same message and is set to operate in the same fashion. Tools used to achieve this standardization include videotapes and course manuals as well as standardized check sheets. These assure that all course materials are identical each time. Without these controls a course can have the same title, but have a different content each time someone new teaches it.

The training at FPL is a unique example of Japanese TQC deployed at a U.S. company. Some think that FPL used TQM management, and, indeed, Mary Walton characterized it as a "Deming management" company in her book on this subject. This is in error. In fact, what was deployed at FPL was Japanese TQC under the direction of Japanese consultants from JUSE, and therein lies a lesson.

Over the period during which TQC was deployed prior to its winning the Deming Prize, FPL charted several indicators of progress and each and every one showed that the company was minimizing problems while maximizing service reliability. Following the award, a management change took place and the new group turned its back on TQC.

At first glance, this may seem surprising since, by winning the Deming Prize, FPL had conclusively proved that TQC would work with U.S. workers and U.S. management—who were properly trained. On polling the new management, however, it decided the workers didn't like TQC.

In the view of many experts, Japanese TQC has a peculiar lack of sensitivity toward certain workers' views, a quality which is apparently tolerable in Japan, but which quickly wears thin here. While TQC is very responsive to business views of the employee, it is indifferent to the integration of the employee's personal life and sensitivities with the business environment. The Japanese corporation offers a job for life, but expects that the employee, in turn, give his or her life to the company. Many people feel that it is only a matter of time before Japanese workers will petition for a review of this policy.

Managers feel the humanistic overtones which Deming emphasizes will save the day. The humanism will keep the workers engaged in the business by involving their concerns as part of the quality effort. This appears to be an absolutely critical embellishment of the TQC process and is fundamental to Deming management and his theory of profound knowledge.

Ranking People

Deming illustrates the issue of artificial scarcity by assuming that human endeavors or abilities may be thought of as being normally distributed. If this is the case, then there is an upper and a lower 5 percent in this, as in any distribution. These are the people out in the ears of the curve. Deming says that in most businesses, 95 percent of the time is spent on these 10 percent of the employees. Half the time is spent figuring out how to keep the superperformers happy, committed, and away from the competition, and the other half is spent on worrying how to make the below average performers more competitive.

Deming makes several points. One way companies deal with the bottom 5 percent is to get rid of it. When they do this, the distribution of abilities and performances simply shifts to the left, resulting in a new bottom 5 percent. Deming believes that all the time spent on ranking people is wasted. This includes annual reviews, class scores, sales goals, and so on. In any group of people, someone will be at the top and someone will be at the bottom. Deming suggests that the review time would be better spent getting everyone to maximize their productivity and not worry about the top and bottom people. This also shifts the company perspective to where it most appropriately belongs, on the majority of the work force—the greatly overlooked middle class.

TEMPERAMENT TESTING

One of the Seven Sages said "Know thyself." This phrase, traced back to ancient Greek literature, has been repeated many times in classical and popular literature. It became the focus of psychotherapy. The message though is always the same: The better people understand themselves, the better they can deal with their interactions with others and with the different situations which life presents.

It has been noted that the Japanese position people in a work situation as if they were different. The Japanese feel that the key to maximizing an individual's productivity, and minimizing friction, is to put the individual with similar types of colleagues. There are two ways this classification could be used. One is if a fully trained technologist presented for a microbiology department position, and tested in such a way that he or she was more appropriate for the serology department. Another is that if four equally qualified individuals presented themselves for the opening in microbiology, the most appropriate personality for that department would be chosen. The question is, what types of tests are used for this classification?

One such test is the Myers-Briggs Type Indicator®.[10] This rather lengthy test is given only by certified psychologists trained in the art. The test was devised by Isabel Myers and her mother Katharine Briggs Myers in the 1950s and was based on Carl Jung's *Psychological Types* published in 1923. A similar classification called the Keirsey Temperament Sorter has recently been published.[11] The four temperament pairs derived from Jung were Introversion (I)/Extroversion (E); Sensation (S)/Intuition (N); Thinking (T)/Feeling (F); and Perceiving (P)/Judging (J). This results in people being classified into 16 different temperament types which are

ISTP	INTP	ISFP	INFP
ISTJ	INTJ	ISFJ	INFJ
ESTJ	ENTJ	ESFJ	ENFJ
ESTP	ENTP	ESFP	ENFP

The classifications are practical in several respects. For instance, although E's are about 75 percent of the population, and I's only 25 percent, both groups derive their restorative energy from quite different sources. I's require solitude to replenish their energy reserves, while E's need the company of others. Recently, I was speaking with the head of human resources for one of the regional operating centers for American Express. This woman appeared extroverted, continually interacting with others in her frequent role as trainer and facilitator. When we spoke of Myers-Briggs testing, she shared with me that she tested as a very polar I. This is a person with a very strong preference for seclusion for revitalization. She remarked that having to go to a party or out dancing after work would be to her like working another eight-hour day. The point is that dancing or partying are considered classical relaxational activities since three-fourths of the population do, in fact, rejuvenate this way. A corollary, though, is that for some people, dancing and partying are real work.

Another practical use of temperament testing is the use of P's and J's in group activities. The P's will never close on an issue. There is never enough data for P's to ever make up their mind. They like the saying, "Statistics is never having to say you're certain." For the P's, there is always the possibility that the next revelation will reverse the present position which they have almost reached. J's are just the opposite. They reach a decision or conclusion very quickly on limited data, which unless they are very bright, or the problem is trivial, will very often be wrong. So for group activities it helps to have a healthy mix of P's and J's in the group. Too many P's, and the issue will never be resolved. Too many J's, and the resolution may not be the right one.

Knowledge of the group's makeup is also helpful for the facilitator. Knowing what types are represented allows the facilitator to recall to task a group of P's who have wandered off on a tangent, or to call for more deliberation in a group of J's who have closed with awesome rapidity on the wrong solution.

Notice that there is no best category. This is simply a way to classify people into broad areas of preference. The practical use of these classifications will depend a great deal on the corporate culture in which the lab operates. I know of one company in which the president has all employees wear name tags which are color coded with the temperament type. An individual can tell at a glance what type is being dealt with. I know other companies in which senior managers will have to be tortured before they ever reveal what type they are. They feel that revealing this will open a window into their soul, and they are accustomed to looking through the one-way glass of the command-and-control type management system. Knowledge is power in this type of setup, and senior management wants to retain all vestiges.

Please explore this area further. Understanding this specialized branch of organizational management can help employees understand job-related, and other social interactions.

Contingency Models of Leadership

Being taught today is an area of discipline variously called organizational behavior, industrial psychology, or, in a TQM setting, an aspect of the voice of the business. This branch of knowledge addresses human activities and the many variables inherent in human activity. TQM management has a general axiom: The more a process depends on people, the more a process needs robustness planning. This is the type of contingency planning that takes into account that a process may show unexpected special variation and designs the process to withstand these vagaries.

Contingency leadership also takes into account that people, as individuals or groups, have behavior variables which influence the success of group activities. Contingency leadership suggests that some variables which affect outcomes are (1) the leaders' personal qualities, (2) the employees' personal qualities, and (3) the groups' traits, attributes, and structure. To assess leadership capability one behavioral psychologist, Fred Fiedler, developed the least preferred co-worker (LPC) test. Leadership candidates are asked to describe a co-worker whom they dislike in terms of friendliness, trustworthiness, consideration, sincerity, and so on through 18 characteristics. If the candidates think that the LPC is very unfriendly, the response is given a high score. If the candidates are more philosophical about it, such that the LPC is perceived as more indifferent than unfriendly perhaps, then the response is given a low score. A high score on the LPC test correlates with a leadership style most comfortable with task-directed leadership. A low score correlates with a leadership style more compatible with group activity. Here, the creativity of the group in conjunction with the leadership will result in the best outcome.

Low scorers on the LPC test don't dislike co-workers all that much. These low scorers are generally well-liked, group-oriented workers. They frequently find themselves promoted into leadership roles because of their popularity. In command-and-control, task-directed operations, they will generally not fair very well, particularly if these are MBO structures where the leaders are left alone to accomplish set goals with little support. They will do quite well in TQM group activities such as quality action teams or project improvement groups. Task teams might be better run by the high scorers on the LPC test if the goals are clear and group input isn't critical to success. The overall message, however, is that people, through these testing activities, get to know themselves and their potential, and get to improve their own capabilities as leaders through this self-awareness.

The Fiedler model of contingency leadership is just one of four models used to assess this aspect of leadership.[12] TQM offers the additional perspective of knowing that the environment in which the leaders operate, the environment structured by management, will be the overriding factor in the leaders' success or failure. For instance, in improving an operation, traditional management thinks of it in terms of getting from here to there. Traditional management thinks in terms of many little tasks which must be accomplished to get there. To this end, traditional managers would prefer a task-oriented leader, and, in fact, a task-oriented leader would do better under this management system. It is when management learns that the more efficient way to get from here to there involves improving the processes involved, and that efficient process improvement requires group input and cooperation, that leaders with different management skills become indispensable.

These are but two examples of a battery of available tests which may help individuals understand themselves in relation to their work environment. In the spirit of TQM these tests are always used in a win-win sense rather than as a purely discriminatory function to sort people.

The Image of the Clinical Laboratory

> On arriving at the party I noticed that many expensive cars were parked out front. "Ah, the surgeons are here," I remarked. I also saw that many Chevys and Fords were there too. "The internists are here also," I observed. Some older cars were parked there also. "The pathologists have arrived," I commented. When I came into the house I saw in the front closet several overshoes. By this I knew that the laboratory men were here as well.

This observation is attributed to William J. Mayo, M.D. (1861–1939).[13] Although the physician's lot seems to have improved in the intervening years, the statement reflects a view of the laboratorian that has not changed much. The laboratory profession, in general, and laboratorians, in particular, suffer from a bad image. This view is reflected not only in the incredible amount of regulation directed at this small segment of the health care field, but also in occasional editorials which reflect on the treatment laboratorians receive in health care settings. These editorials generally reflect on lack of respect and a general underappreciation of the contribution of laboratorians to the health care process.

For instance, in the February 1992 issue of *Medical Laboratory Observer*, an author suggests the name clinical laboratory scientist to replace lab technician or technologist. The purpose was to suggest a degree of sophistication which the name scientist would bring. In today's society, however, scientists are popularly portrayed as individuals removed from society's goals and more concerned with their own private interests. This is reflected in the archetypical mad scientist, in movies like *Revenge of the Nerds* in which today's teenagers are portrayed as unusual if they happen to be interested in science.

This is remarkable inasmuch as laboratorians frequently have education and training equal to anyone on the hospital staff, up to and including the administrators. Laboratorians may have completed a four-year technical baccalaureate degree which, by any measure, is a real accomplishment. Why then the feeling that the laboratory, among hospital departments, is held in low regard?

To better understand this I believe the field of cultural and behavioral anthropology should be discussed. This science examines human behavior at the most basic level. This is the level at which society developed expectations over many years of evolution and during which society grew larger and more complex. Society's expectations for its members evolved as well.

For years cultural anthropologists thought that the main characteristic that separated humans from the rest of the animal kingdom was speech. Then after it was found that Washoe, Nim Chimpsky, and other chimpanzees could handle Ameslan reasonably well, it was decided that it wasn't speech after all, but tool use that conveyed humanity. Subsequently, the scientists discovered that, when they needed to, the animals could routinely use tools in some cases better than the scientists could after considerable practice. In one case, an anthropologist was never able to duplicate a primate's use of sticks to pull termites out of a mound, even after months of practice. Subsequently, when it was determined that humans share 95 percent of their DNA with chimpanzees, it began to appear that perhaps humans differed only in degree and not in kind from the rest of the animal world.

Scientists now suggest that it is altruism that is the chief characteristic which truly helps differentiate human beings from other animals and mammals. Through this, humans are able to project the consequences of their actions on others, and to make their responses more suitable for society's benefit by putting self-interests as a lessor priority. The playwright turned cultural anthropologist Robert Ardrey thought he had found an example of altruism in the wild when he noticed that Thompson gazelles would leap up in the air rather than run away when a pack of African hunting dogs came over the hill after the gazelles. Ardrey believed, this unusual action, called stotting, was the jumping gazelles' way of warning the herd of an impending attack, a truly altruistic act. The sensible and self-serving thing would have been to run away and save themselves first.

On later analysis, it was found that the jumping gazelles were, in fact, letting the dogs know that they were the healthiest, most fit, and the hardest to run down. Thus, if the dogs wanted an easy meal, they might want to chase after the young and the infirm, which on even closer analysis, was exactly what the dogs had always been doing.

When applying the principles of altruism to the health care field, the public expects that health care providers will exhibit this highest, most compassionate, and humanistic virtue of altruism. The public's expectations are met in the image of the hospital as an institution for making sick people well. The public's expectations are again met in the image of the nurses, doctors, and support departments whose role is to make patients well.

These expectations are not met in the role of the lab, which is to analyze patients. These expectations are particularly not met with the independent, or reference lab, which exists outside the hospital setting and which unfortunately may be viewed as a business which derives income at the expense of the sick.

Some journalists and politicians have exploited the public's view of the lab for personal self-interest, and together they are responsible for CLIA '88. No other legislation in the past year even came close to attracting the number of comments that CLIA did. The only legislation that generated comparable excitement happened several years ago when the tax code was revised to delete certain write-offs to which U.S. business had become firmly attached, such as the business lunch and the free car.

The amount of attention that labs get is unrelated to their fiscal impact on health care spending. This is clearly evidenced by comparing total health care costs with the lab contribution to those costs.

In 1990, U.S. health care expenditures reached $666.2 billion. The laboratory contribution to this figure was about 4.5 percent. In effect, if all the laboratories were closed completely, hospital, independent, physician owned, and so on, the taxpayers would save less than a nickel on their health care tax dollar.

Clearly then, the government would benefit taxpayers by adopting Pareto techniques and prioritizing regulatory efforts to focus on the predominant root causes of health care spending, rather than using the lab as a red herring continually dragged across the public path. This diverts attention from the fact that the government has consistently been unwilling to identify and control principal sources of health care spending and unable to provide leadership out of the health care crisis.

In this way also, the government would cease trying to capitalize on an inequitable lab image which its actions help foster. The way out of this situation is to follow Deming's advice. Indeed, it takes a much deeper knowledge to run a business or a government well, and that the community must recognize that laboratorians are educated, skilled, intelligent, and hard-working people that contribute professionally to health care and do so in a very cost-effective way.

External and Internal Motivation

Deming spends a great deal of time on the concept of internal motivation. External motivation he views as the traditional ways in which companies encourage acceptable performance or discourage unacceptable achievement by employees. He believes this convention will, at best, result in zero-defect mentality in workers. In effect, they will deliver what the company has outlined as specifications for productivity.

Deming believes that a better way would be to install systems which would encourage continual improvement of the workers and their group: a continual reduction in error and process variation and a continual increase in productivity. Deming feels this will only come about from the energy that comes from people who have bought into the TQM philosophy and are empowered and enabled to make their contributions in a participatory way. They will also realize dignity and self-esteem in the process.[14]

In summary Deming says,[14]

> The transformation will take us into a new system of reward. We must restore the individual, and do so in the complexities of interactions with the rest of the world. The transformation will release the power of human resource contained in intrinsic motivation. In place of competition for high rating, high grades, to be number one, there will be cooperation on problems of common interest between people, divisions, companies, governments, and countries. The result will, in time, be greater innovation, applied science, technology, expansion of the market, greater service, and greater material reward for everyone. There will be joy in work, and joy in learning. Anyone that enjoys his work is a pleasure to work with. Everyone will win and no one will lose.

NOTES

1. W. Edwards Deming, "Foundation for Management in the Western World." A paper delivered at the Institute of Management Sciences, Osaka, Japan, July 24, 1989. Revised April 1, 1990 and available from W. Edwards Deming, Ph.D., Consultant in Statistical Studies, 4924 Butterworth Pl., Washington, D.C. 20016; 202-363-8552.

2. Ibid.

3. Alfie Kohn, *No Contest—The Case Against Competition* (Boston: Houghton Mifflin, 1986).

4. Howard and Shelly Gitlow and Alan and Rosa Oppenheim, *Tools and Methods for the Improvement of Quality* (Homewood, Ill.: Richard D. Irwin, 1989).

5. Masaaki Imai. *Kaizen: The Key to Japan's Competitive Success* (New York: Random House, 1986), 26–27.

6. Anne H. Rosenfeld, *Archaeology of Affect* (Washington, D.C.: National Institute of Mental Health, National Institutes of Health, 1976). This is a review of Paul MacLean's work.

7. Roger W. Sperry, "Lateral Specialization of Cerebral Function in the Surgically Separated Hemispheres," in F. J. McGuigan and R. A. Schoonover, eds., *The Psychophysiology of Thinking* (New York: Academic Press, 1973): pp. 209–229.

8. Shintiro Ishihara, *The Japan That Can Say No* (New York: Simon & Schuster, 1989), 91–93.

9. Deborah Tannen, Ph.D., *You Just Don't Understand* (New York: Ballantine, 1991), 282.

10. Myers-Briggs Type Indicator® and MBTI® are registered trademarks of Consulting Psychologists Press, Inc., Palo Alto, Calif.

11. David Keirsey and Marilyn Bates, *Please Understand Me*, 5th ed. (Del Mar, Calif., Prometheus Nemesis Book Co., 1984).

12. Don Hellriegel, John W. Slocum, Jr., and Richard Woodman, *Organizational Behavior*, 6th ed. (New York: West Publishing Co., 1992), 396.

13. *Macmillan Dictionary of Quotations*. (New York: Macmillan Publishing, 1987), 164.

14. See note 1.

3

Sources of Lab Error

INTRODUCTION

The conventional picture generally portrayed of testing in a clinical laboratory is people and machines making numbers. For instance, a myopic view of the generation of a glucose value is a technologist and a glucose machine. The scenario includes the technologist aspirating the patient sample, putting it in the machine, and reading a glucose value. When things go wrong, blame the tech.

It is known, however, that if a tech injects 20 sequential samples of the same specimen into the machine, the values will vary somewhat. They will actually be a set of values called a distribution. The values will be distributed around a mean value. This gives the first clue that this process of running a glucose has some built-in variability.

An additional perspective is that no matter how hard the tech tries, how good the tech's intentions are, how well trained and educated the tech is, the same value cannot be generated 20 times in a row. Whose fault is that? The tech and the machine represent a two-part system, and the combination of their output has some built-in variability. It should already be evident that the system output and the series of glucose values are not entirely under the tech's control. Perhaps then, when something goes wrong the tech cannot always be blamed. Then again, how often can the tech be blamed?

The Centers for Disease Control and Prevention (CDC) published the results of a literature survey of 800 publications related to lab error. Two studies indicate that errors associated with the technical analysis (analytical error) of a proficiency testing sample are responsible for wrong results only about one-third of the time.[1]

This must mean then that the system for generating lab results is much more extensive than just the tech and the machine. The tech-machine component, although significant, results in only a minor contribution to overall error. In fact, the system can be traced from the patient to the specimen to transportation to analysis to reporting; and in each one of these component processes, there is opportunity for error.

Look at the error components associated with the patient. In a hospital situation, the patient may not have checked in yet when timed testing is ordered. Or the patient may be in the hospital but unavailable due to another procedure being performed, which will influence other lab tests. Or the patient may be overhydrated, underhydrated, nonfasting, taking drugs that interfere with certain lab tests, supine, or upright. Or it may be at a time of day which is a peak or a trough of the analyte variability.

The same sort of analysis can be done for the potential error contributions to each of the systems making up the overall process. From this, it is easily seen that the overall system is quite extensive, and that there may be many error components not at all under the control of the lab.

TQM, however, adopts a position of much greater perspective than even this. TQM refers to an extended system in which the responsibility for lab results includes the effect of the facility executive management environment in which the laboratory resides. This would include the ability of the executive management system to provide a vision and mission for the hospital and the lab. It would include the management system's involvement in planning to include establishing and meeting departmental needs for personnel, their training, education, and job enrichment, and the equipment to meet the facility's mission. It would include management involvement for establishing systems of feedback where the voice of the lab and other departments could be heard down to the level of the individual employee. Thus, process improvement could include input from people actually doing the processes. It would include establishing a management information system so that the proper data could be collected and organized to analyze progress. It would include a cross-functional control and communication system to coordinate interdepartmental activities in establishing and meeting quality goals. None of these components is under the technologist's or even the laboratory's control. They are all a responsibility of the facility's executive management.

THE SYSTEMS APPROACH TO THE LABORATORY OPERATION

The systems approach to maximizing reliability is based on the teachings of Deming, Juran, Shewhart, Edwards, and others. They recommend treating operational processes as systems and explain that the variability in these systems is the source of error.

Figure 3.1 is an integrated flowchart which shows the laboratory as the system, with specimens coming in and reports going out. The inherent error of such a system is comprised of many diverse components, and a badly designed lab process will result in a high reporting error. It must be recognized that the reliability of such a system can never rise above the latent error or design error inherent in the system and its component processes. Conversely, as the reliability of the component processes is improved, the overall system reliability improves according to well-known rules of probability.

SPECIAL AND COMMON CAUSES OF VARIABILITY

Common-cause variation is the variation inherent to the system. It is the noise or intrinsic variability within which the process operates and delivers whatever service or product the process provides. Common-cause variation is a limiting factor, and the process delivery can only be as good as its basic design, and can only be improved by improving the process design. The main difference between the two sources of process variation is that common-cause variation is always the responsibility of management. The degree of common-cause variation exists because of management's design of the system, it remains because of management's maintenance of the system, and it will only be lessened or improved when management steps in and changes the system.

For example, if new techs are routinely undertrained, then their lack of seasoning may affect their results. It is management's responsibility for training, as well as retraining and the associated documentation. If the machine is not routinely maintained, again the results may be affected. And again, although it may be the tech's responsibility to actually do the maintenance, it is a management responsibility to see that a schedule is set and that the work is routinely done. If this involves a maintenance contract, and the option for accepting or rejecting it is done at a higher level based on financial constraints, this may not even be under lab control. The lab will catch the heat, though, if the test results don't go out.

Special cause variation is everything else that can affect the system which is not a routine part of the system. This is an important distinction,

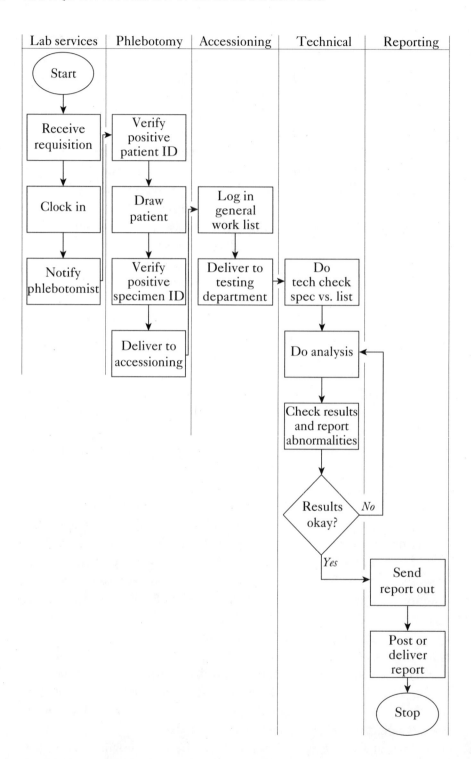

Figure 3.1: The laboratory diagnostic system. Flowchart of a typical laboratory analytical process.

because special variation is removed by analysis of its causes and special remediation is taken to prevent its recurrence. This may be done by and under the control of the system operators. Special variation is said to have an assignable cause. The reason the differentiation is important is because workers are frequently blamed for common-cause problems, over which they have no control. Special-cause variation would be if an outdated or incorrect reagent were used in the machine. The cause is assignable to the wrong reagent, and it is correctable and controllable by the line operator. Other assignable causes relate to the myriad of things that can affect a human operator, which are not management controllable, and over which the operator does have control. Human variability, however, is a distinct topic because humans are, to an extent, slightly different each day of their lives due to experiences undergone the day before. So it is important that process design take into account this ingredient. This is addressed later under the topic of robustness planning.

Juran estimates that common-cause variability accounts for about 80 percent of process problems. This has given rise to the Juran 80/20 rule, which states that 80 percent of the problems in a system are due to 20 percent of the causes. A corollary, according to Juran, is that operators only have about 20 percent controllability of their system and the remainder is under management control. Deming estimates management control as high as 96 percent while Ishikawa approximates it at 66 percent. There is clearly room for some personal bias in interpreting what data are available, but the experts are unanimous in according management the lion's share of the accountability and virtually all of the responsibility for effecting improvement in systems which show only common-cause variability.

Figure 3.2 summarizes these thoughts. Note that a system can be thought to consist of six parts—human resources, machine, method, measurement, materials, and environment. These are used in systems analysis to study and eliminate process variation. The special-cause variation in a system must be eliminated before a good statistical study can be done. With only common-cause variation, the system is said to be in a state of statistical control.

In principal, a system must be under statistical control before a valid statistical analysis can be done and conclusions drawn from it. If special- or assignable-cause variability is still inherent to the process, then the statistical analysis can still be done, but the results must be interpreted with great care by someone who is very skilled in the art. To illustrate these concepts, the next section looks at an accounting function in a hospital setting. In order to measure the effectiveness of the accounting system, it first had to be stabilized and the special variation had to be removed prior to further analysis. Deming calls this the SDCA cycle, in which the S stands for standardize.

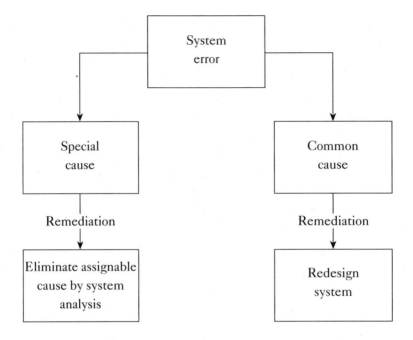

Figure 3.2: System error. The system or process is divided into the two main components of special and common cause. Minimizing the contribution of each of these causes, or remediation, is quite different for each as shown.

SYSTEM STABILIZATION

Figure 3.3 shows a flowchart of an accounts payable (AP) system in a hospital setting. The AP group wanted to keep good relationships with their suppliers, and so it decided to track its responsiveness to invoices related to supplier services. It turned out, however, that the system had some built-in variability which needed addressing before this could happen. In the system as initially studied, the department managers would request a product service or, in some cases, facilities work which was done by outside suppliers. Some time after the work was complete, the managers would get called by the supplier who would ask when it would be paid. The department managers never knew the answer because the system never had them in the information loop after the request for payment was generated by the managers and sent to accounts payable. The managers didn't know whether their request for payment had been received, and if it had been received, whether accounting was going to pay immediately or put the account on a future payment line.

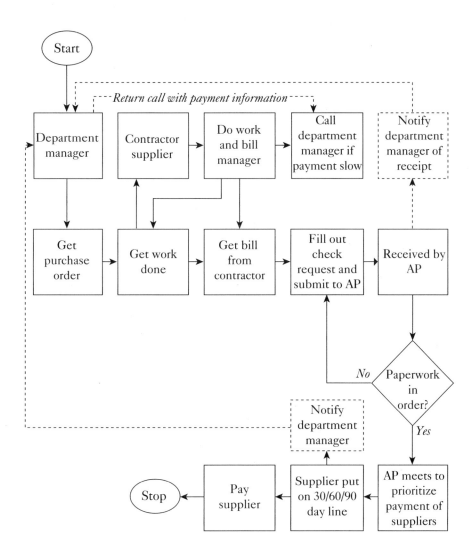

Figure 3.3: An accounts payable system—SDCA method. In this accounts payable system, the initial process is shown by the solid lines. Suppliers were prioritized for payment without the knowledge of the department that originally ordered the work, product, or service. When the supplier called the department manager for information on payment, the manager had no idea whether the payment request had been received by accounts payable or when accounting was going to generate payment. The process improvement is shown by the dotted lines in which the department is notified of the receipt of request and the payment schedule.

Since the calls from suppliers were a nuisance, which the department managers wanted no part of, some of the less-tolerant managers switched their ordering techniques to another path which the accounts payable system accommodated. They requested payment up front for the services prior to rendering. This resulted in the hospital being put in a position where it continually had cash going out for services it hadn't yet received. The managers, on the other hand, were happy because the supplier calls for payment stopped.

This system runs counter to the concept of just-in-time (JIT) purchasing which is designed to reduce inventories so that the hospital doesn't have large sums of cash tied up in stored inventory. The JIT concept would prescribe that the departments work with the AP group to assure that suppliers were being paid promptly, but only on conclusion of delivery.

A solution was reached in which the AP department notified the department managers upon receipt of the request for payment and also on the supplier payment schedule. The pay-in-advance option was deleted, except in construction contracts which called for a percentage up front. Thus the department managers had the information they needed to handle the requests, and the company's cash flow schedule was eased by paying for services conventionally, that is, when rendered. In addition, AP now had control over payment to suppliers and could now reliably track its own efforts at improving the customer–supplier relationship.

This is an example of the standardize-do-check-act (SDCA) cycle. The process was improved simply by finding the best process and stabilizing it. Frequently, in systems analysis, cases like this occur in which a better method is found in a simple fashion. This doesn't mean that this process cannot be improved by a more thorough analysis, but the major improvement was easily done in keeping with TQM principles. The stabilized system, free of special variation, could now be subjected to routine statistical analysis, and further improved, if necessary, using techniques related to the PDCA cycle.

OTHER TYPES OF SYSTEMS

To gain more appreciation for the systems concept, a few examples of nonlaboratory systems may help.

A company had recently finished construction of an elevated train transport system including about 45 miles of track on top of concrete supports separated by inverted U-shaped concrete supports. The track was about 25 feet from the ground, and the construction involved planting the supports, laying the concrete track bed on top of them, and then laying the track on top of that. A great deal of construction, then, was done about 25 feet above the ground.

Many workers fell from the construction site and suffered injuries typical of that sort of fall including damage to the cervical vertebrae. Not only is the quality of the workers' life greatly diminished, but this is also an expensive type of injury requiring lifelong maintenance—sometimes even in a respirator. The system was a construction project designed to build an elevated transport system, and as one of the common causes of variation, workers got hurt which is not only uncaring, but also expensive.

It is important to identify the system and the desired system output. Without specifying that the system is designed to lay track in a safe fashion, it is possible to view the system as being comprised of components, one of which is to injure workers. In fact, a construction system with no restraints like this one will injure people on a fairly reliable and predictable basis.

In this example, the workers falling could have been considered special cause by management. Its remedy would have been to hire less clumsy people or embark on an enhanced training program designed to give the construction workers the grace and high-wire capabilities of circus acrobats. Well, acrobats still fall, and the fact that it took a system design change to eliminate the problem is the key to identifying it as common-cause variation, and thus, out of the operators' control as far as remediation is concerned.

Recent construction safety practices in elevated environments now include safety gear such as that used by mountaineers. Workers are issued harnesses with a line and a clip, something akin to the safety lines that mariners use to maneuver on pitching decks in rough seas. The cost of this gear is more than offset by the savings attributable to the convalescence of injured workers.

This is a system redesign. It is an example of designing for a quality outcome. It is in keeping with Deming's statement "cease reliance on final inspection." Deming is fond of saying that management by outcome will result in a bad outcome. He likens this to driving while looking in the rearview mirror and asks how soon one will crash. If a product is made wrong, it can be scrapped or reworked, both expensive actions which can be avoided with proper system design. When workers fall, as in the example, they can be buried or fixed, again outcomes which can be avoided by proper design. Managing by outcome puts the company in a reflexive mode—constantly reacting to events. Managing by design for quality puts the company in charge of its own destiny.

Many years ago, U.S. steel mills moved large quantities of molten steel by having the almost white-hot liquid in a large cauldron or in a ladle with a lip on it for pouring the tons of molten metal. With all the catwalks and overhead cranes that surrounded the work area there was plenty of opportunity to fall in and workers occasionally did.

When this happened, the vat of steel was always discarded. This wasn't entirely a humanitarian gesture, because the carbon content of steel causes it to become more brittle. With all the carbon in the human body the steel was made too brittle for further use such as cold rolling into sheets or bar stock. Now in modern Japanese steel plants, overheads, catwalks, and conveyor belts are located where people don't pass under or over, as is now the case in this country. Note that the solution was to remove common-cause variation by redesigning the system, not by teaching people to walk a tightrope.

Another example of a system involves an incident at Los Angeles International Airport in February of 1991. Here a bewildered air traffic controller landed a 737 jet on top of a smaller commuter plane on the same runway getting ready for takeoff. The flight safety record of the airlines is widely used as an example of a six-sigma operation, and when something like this happens, it is widely studied and the lessons learned are incorporated into future systems designed at preventing a recurrence.

The flight controller was unable to see the commuter aircraft because her view was blocked, and due to equipment restrictions, she was unable to physically move to a point with a better view. The system within which she was working was designed to ensure that aircraft would land and take off safely.

In this case, a pair of backup precautions, which were supposed to be part of the operation design, were not in place. An electronic indicator designed to tell the controller if a plane was on one of the runways was broken and had not been repaired. Further, although a second controller had been mandated by the FAA, this person had not yet been hired. Had this person been available, he or she could have gone around the viewing obstruction and checked the location of the commuter plane. In other words, a system had been designed to provide sufficient safeguards, but the system wasn't followed.

These safeguards are referred to as redundant operations and are widely used in attempts to foolproof an operation. Redundancy is used frequently in the clinical lab where assay results are run with multiple controls and reviewed by senior personnel before release. Abnormals are rerun.

Engineers are careful of how they apply redundancy. For instance, in a fighter aircraft the pilot has a control stick which is attached to the horizontal stabilizer in the tail of the airplane. If the plane is shot at by ground fire or in air combat, the control cable, which connects the stick in the cockpit to the tail surface, can be severed. Thus, it makes sense to connect the two points by several cables, or, as in modern times, by no cables at all but by remote sensors and servos. These are redundant engineering designs striving to make certain that a single lucky shot doesn't make the whole aircraft uncontrollable. These are good and they work.

As another example, in pumping a ship bilge dry, a large pump, designed to last a long time, can be used. If this single pump fails in a storm, however, the ship can fill with water and founder. So, in principal, it might appear to be wiser to use two smaller pumps, so that when one fails the other can take over. The problem with this is that when the first pump goes bad, the second one is called into play using a sensor which has only one seldom-used function; this is to detect the failure of the first pump and kick in the second one. The problem is that the sensor can fail and the redundancy becomes unavailable. The sensor is a weak link. In addition, the backup pump may not start because it has never been used and may not have been maintained for the long period of time since installation. A good engineer won't use this type of redundancy without specifying a corresponding rigorous preventive maintenance protocol.

Returning to the case of the air traffic controller, a typical American management reaction would have been one of assigning blame to the controller. Thus, remediation would have been in the form of warnings, retraining, probation, and the like.

A Japanese manager, on the other hand, would have apologized to the controller for putting her in a position where this sort of outcome could occur. Gitlow and Gitlow, in *The Deming Guide to Quality and Competitive Position*, describe a 1985 incident involving Japan Airlines in which a 747 crashed causing 520 deaths. The CEO of the airline subsequently resigned following this event, thus acknowledging the culpability of top management. In other words, Japanese management accepts responsibility for the outcome of system failures, as is proper, since it is also responsible for design, deployment, and compliance of the quality management effort.

According to Ishihara, in his book *The Japan That Can Say No*, the crash of the 747 was the fault of Boeing's shoddy workmanship. Four employees were responsible, and Boeing admitted the employees' error. The plane had been damaged in a hard landing, and the repairs called for a splice plate to be riveted between bulkheads. The Boeing people inserted the bolts so that they only went through two of the three thicknesses. The section broke loose, and when it did, it damaged the hydraulic system causing the pilots to lose control and crash. Ishihara says that, "Such shoddy performance by a Japanese corporation is unthinkable." The fact that the CEO resigned, however, shows how deeply the responsibility is felt at that level. The CEO thought that his people should have caught Boeing's mistake.

Deming says, "The quality of an organization is limited by the quality of its top management. The company can be no better than these people."

OPERATOR CONTROL

Juran says a defect is under operator control if the operators know what they are supposed to be doing, what they are actually doing, and if they have a means of regulating their own performance. If these three criteria are not met then the defect is under management control. If the operators precipitate the fault in the case where they are not in control, they are simply the means to the defect and not the cause of it. In controllability studies, data indicate that about 80 percent of these problems are under management control and only about 20 percent are due to operator error.

In the case of the LAX air traffic accident, the one person to hold blameless is the controller. She acted in accord with expected behavior of an individual trapped in a well-designed but badly deployed system. She was subject to too much input. Further, the lack of backup in the system wasn't of her doing or under her control.

Deming's red bead experiment is his powerful example of a system which is not under the employees' control, but for which they are nonetheless held responsible. In a variation of this, personnel pick marbles out of a box which contains an equal number of red and black balls. After nine choices or so, the people with more black balls than red get fired.

Examine both of these examples in terms of zero-defect management. Zero-defect management has as a central tenet the admonition, "do it right the first time, every time, all the time." If this is used to control the elevated rail construction project, then the supervisor concentrates on training people not to fall off, and posts signs like, "Don't fall off the tracks." In Deming's view this is like holding up a sign to a thundercloud, "Don't rain on me." If you don't want to get wet, then put up a roof. If you don't want workers to fall, tie them up there with safety harnesses.

Consider redundancy as it relates to transportation systems. Redundancy is applied to enhance the reliability of a system. If the system doesn't particularly require great reliability, then the cost may simply not be justified. For example, in a bus there is one driver. If the engine catches fire the driver pulls the bus over to the side and everyone gets off. With any luck the damage to life and property won't be too bad.

In an airliner, there are now not one but two people driving. If a plane engine catches fire, it is the copilot's job to fly out of it while the pilot effects a fix and directs strategy. The idea is to buy time in order for the copilot to pull it over and park it, because if the copilot can't, then everyone has pretty well had it. This is the application of reliability proportional to how bad it is needed. In a troubled airliner, reliability is needed very badly indeed. In the bus, perhaps not so much.

For instance, if the system is a lift operator moving TV sets in a warehouse, then training and possibly some foolproofing systems are needed. Foolproofing might include setting the jaws of the squeeze so that the sets can't be crushed, because if the operator errs, then a set is dropped or squashed. If a flight controller errs, the plane may land in the middle of an interstate. See the difference? More reliability is needed in the second instance, and both cases can forget about zero defects and concentrate on system design for an optimized outcome, with maximum reliability consistent with cost and safety considerations.

Examine the same two examples in terms of MBO. Recall Deming's principle 11 which advises to "eliminate management by numerical goals." The LAX control tower supervisor may have had as a goal the operation of the tower with one controller. This is an example of a goal set in keeping with short-term economic constraints, but inconsistent with quality and reliability as shown by outcome measures.

In the construction example, the goal may have been so many miles of track a day, which might have been slowed by hooking and unhooking harnesses. In both of these examples, the goals are met in keeping with internal costs, which then are more than offset later by external costs. This is the false economy which seems to be so little realized in most current management schemes but which is the crux of Japanese TQC.

Figure 3.4 shows how the laboratory can be viewed as being comprised of many subsystems representing subsidiary operations. In applying TQM methods to these systems or operations it is important to delineate which part of the overall system is under study. If it is the courier system for instance, this process is isolated and techniques, which will be described

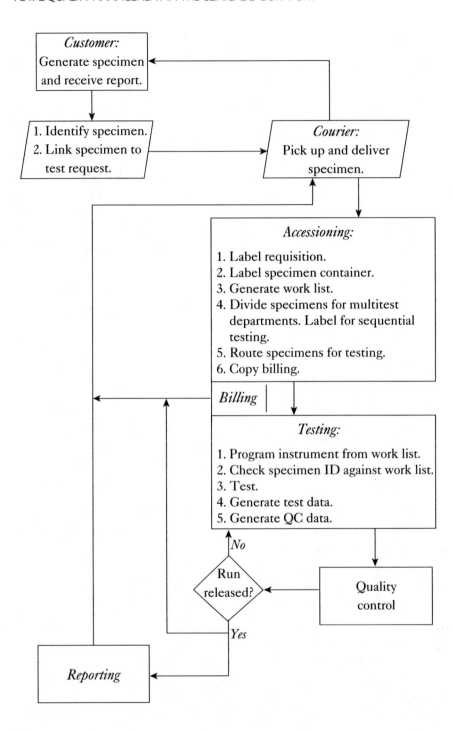

Figure 3.4: Reference laboratory system flowchart.

later, are applied. The system shown is an outreach lab or independent lab and is basically a cyclical system, roughly in the shape of a figure 8, with the couriers at the intersection of the upper and lower balls of the 8.

In this manner, each system has a source of supply prior to its function, and the customer is the next operation in the overall lab system. This customer's requirements define the minimum quality aspects of that system's function. Then the analysis for optimizing the system can be applied to a rather small portion of the total operation or to a larger piece.

Deming says of Japan, "The boundaries to the system are the boundaries of the country." Actually it goes far beyond this since the Japanese and their TQC-based business management system appear virtually around the world.

Variation in these systems results in error. And so, understanding the sources of variation and methods of minimizing variation of the system are cardinal aims of TQM. Variation has many sources and components. Understanding what these are, and the manner in which they may be remedied, are the next steps in understanding how TQM can fit into the lab operation.

HUMAN ERROR

Just as process variability can be broken down into special and common cause, the human component of this variability can be dissected out and analyzed. Figure 3.5 compares human error to system error by dividing human error into special and common cause.

Recognizing that human error has two separate sources helps in understanding the strategies used to diminish it. Juran originally divided human error into two major classes, technique error and inadvertent error. This captures the essence of the special- and common-cause classification. Juran, however, also added deliberate error. This type of error was called sabotage during World War II, but Juran also includes bias or coloration in this class. This special-cause error is witting, intentional, and consistent. He feels that another potential cause of human error is misinterpretation. This, however, would be under the category of a system error since operators can't remediate on their own without supervisory intervention. Irrespective of this, the two major contributors can still be considered common cause, or random error associated with the system limits, and special cause, or error associated with things that could conceivably be fixed.

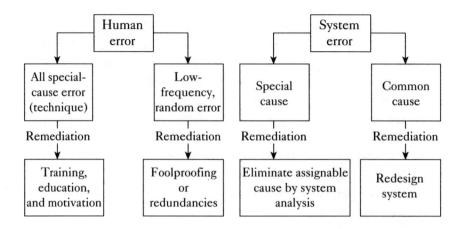

Figure 3.5: Comparing human error to system error. The comparison of human error to system error is shown with remedial techniques. Although common-cause error can be lowered in the ordinary system by redesigning the system, the human analogue of common-cause error, the low-frequency random error which remains after the worker's technique is perfect cannot be eliminated by redesign. The worker cannot be redesigned, and so redundant or foolproofing measures are used instead.

Recall that the common-cause error can only be reduced by addressing the system limits which are inherent in its design. Special-cause error, on the other hand, can be reduced by operator training, education, instrument calibration, and preventive maintenance, proper use of controls, and motivational techniques. Various incentive and reward programs also affect the operators' ability to perform.

Most important is the degree of operator control. Juran feels that in a company run by conventional management about 80 percent of abatable error is caused by management and not by operators. Accordingly, it is necessary for supervisors to examine the process for which the operators are responsible and to make certain that the control of the process is within the domain of the operators. Thus, improving the operators will, in fact, result in a net improvement of the process.

The game of golf provides a good illustration of error that is responsive to incentive and that which isn't. Regardless of how people feel about golf, most people understand it as a game in which players stand on a tee and hit a ball onto the green. If the hole is short, this can be done with one stroke.

Imagine a typical Sunday golfer standing on a tee, looking across a small lake to the green on the other side. On a good day, given 10 balls, this golfer can hit seven on the green, two in the vicinity of the green, and one in the water.

Now suppose you are the coach and it is your job to better performance or lower the error rate. Try doubling the salary. Deming quotes the head of GM saying "If we doubled the salary of everyone in the plant, the error rate tomorrow would be the same as today." This is an astute observation. Deming prefers nonmonetary rewards as an integral part of an ongoing program designed to enhance joy in the workplace. Certainly pleasant surroundings help lead to good morale which, in turn, puts employees in the fitting frame of mind for quality production.

Golfers, though, seem happy enough being where they are. In effect they are cheerful temporary employees of the golf course, and their job is to get around the course with as few strokes as possible. That is their quality goal, and it is the same as their production goal.

Return to the Sunday golfer. The offer of a large cash incentive, or alternatively, punishment and humiliation, will not result in any great difference in performance. In other words, the golfer is immune to incentive techniques, either the carrot or the stick. This is an important lesson in management. Managers waste a lot of time trying to get employees to do better using incentive techniques. Most error isn't responsive to incentive routines.

Training and education of the Sunday golfers will undoubtedly improve their game, and how much depends on their innate capabilities. People are different. Good coaching, though, will unquestionably improve all but the most intractable game. Having done this though, you, as the coach, will reach another plateau, limited by the performance ability of the subject. From the job standpoint, if this is good enough, then great. If not, the Sunday golfers must be replaced by professionals. This is a system change, a system redesign. The limit of the system performance had been reached by optimizing the capabilities of the Sunday golfers, and special variation had been minimized. Better performance needs the professionals.

These professionals may now be able to hit 10 out of 10 balls onto the green virtually every time. Conventionally a hole like this is called a par three. It is expected that, on the average, a good player will hit the ball on the green and use two putts to get it in the hole. The allowable system variation defining acceptable performance specifies one to three shots for this type of hole.

Application of Japanese TQC would require that acceptable performance be one shot, each and every time. Remember that the purpose is to get the ball in the hole, not just on the green. Since players couldn't perform this reliably, they would be better replaced by a machine that could. This is also a key point and is incorporated in the lab from bar code reading for positive sample identification to robotics.

Perhaps at some point the laboratory will become a robotic environment. It is certainly on its way. Nissan built a plant in Smyrna, Tennessee which is largely robotic, and the human employees mind the machines. This is not too distant from the current state of affairs in the clinical lab where, other than specimen preparation and reporting, the machines do the majority of the work except perhaps in certain low-volume areas. With the human component removed, reliability of a system becomes easy to analyze and predict.

The Japanese view the most important function of the human resources department as getting people working together who are most suited to one another from the standpoint of personality, common interests, and general point of view. The Japanese view credentials as secondary to the ability to get along in a team fashion.

This emphasizes the team approach which the Japanese view as so vital to their technique, and which is so secondary in the United States. In this country, some view the team approach as subjugating individuality and creativity, aspects which have always rated high here. A lesson from the Japanese system is that shifting priorities of the human resource department can result in unexpected dividends, if the management structure can foster group creativity while not restricting individual contribution.

MAXIMIZING HUMAN PRODUCTIVITY

In the system approach just reviewed, all error components can be improved by similar techniques. Human error, however, is a particularly difficult subject to handle by itself. Put differently, in analyzing error components, the human contribution is the most difficult to deal with in a consistent manner. This is because it is difficult to determine when individuals are performing at maximum error-free productivity without pushing them past that limit. Exceeding that limit will result in increased error in their work. After an operator has been overstressed, it is possible to determine where the break point occurred.

This is an important corollary because, in practice, this is exactly the way operator capability is determined. So then even the traditional practice of modern management styles may result in overstressing personnel. This can result from the overzealous application of corrective methods. Once workers reach the limit of remediation, the random inherent error or noise in the human work process is encountered. This must be addressed by system redesign.

Recognizing that these two very different error components exist, however, will help managers understand that there are limiting results to be derived from continual pressure to perform and that at some point the system will have to be redesigned if any improvement is to occur. This redesign may incorporate a system of additional review in keeping with the critical nature of the process. This approach can result in error reduction consistent with any set goal.

PHYSIOLOGICAL BASIS FOR HUMAN OPERATOR ERROR

Understanding the physiological basis for human error is important because there is a point at which the analogy between common cause removal by system redesign breaks down with regard to workers. Conceptually, a system may be endlessly improved and the mechanical components endlessly perfected. With the human analogue, however, one eventually is faced with the human unit, the employee. Since the employee cannot be redesigned, as the golf analogy showed, it is best to understand the underlying components of human nature, thus emphasizing system design in keeping with human strengths and weaknesses.

Recent research in human behavior indicates that humans initially act involuntarily, and that conscious action has already been reviewed once by a higher functional area of the brain. This is rather counterintuitive since human beings all feel that they act consciously after more or less careful consideration of the contemplated act.

Dr. Richard Restak in his book *The Brain* reviews the work done by the founder of this research area, Dr. Emanuel Donshin. He worked under a Department of Defense grant and was asked to evaluate military leadership potential. Donshin claims that it is possible to discern when an urge to act reaches the brain processing centers and relates that interaction with conscious movement. By means of electroencephalography, Donshin characterizes what he refers to as the p300 wave. This wave is the brain neuropotential which indicates conscious thought.

If human subjects randomly look at a set of cards and are told to raise their right hand every time an ace comes up, the study shows that the muscle response precedes the conscious thought to move the hand. When the subjects see the ace, the potential to fire the muscle accrues before they consciously decide to do it. This overriding conscious review is quantifiable as Donshin's p300 frontal lobe potential. This appears to be excess evolutionary baggage which human beings have carried over the years. At one time this response had a very real survival value. Early in human development, on the savannah perhaps, it might have been advantageous to act first and think later. Even now human beings carry the fight or flight response which more than one public speaker has encountered on stage.

In the insect world, one of the best survivors is the common household cockroach. A truly ancient bug, the roach has on its back a set of hairs which are connected directly to the legs. The hairs sense movement and when someone tries to swat the roach, the wave from the paper pressure front is received by the hairs and sets the legs directly in motion. Whether the roach ever consciously reviews this with an accompanying p300 wave is unknown. But in essence the roach is off and running before it is aware of it, and has survived over the aeons because of this response.

In the human arena Dr. Donshin observes, "A person who reacts prior to the p300 response, is acting impulsively, will make more errors, and generally will be a poor choice as a leader." Parenthetically, however, this person might make a fine roach.

When children play "Simon Says" or "Mother May I," they are trying to get their opponents to react prior to the p300 wave. In so many words, they try to get their opponents to act before they think.

In his book *The Emperor's New Mind*, Roger Penrose reviews related experiments and arrives at a similar conclusion. It, however, includes reflexive responses, such as those used by table tennis players or combat jet pilots. These are not characterized as well, but Penrose feels that they may be similarly involved in introducing low-level random error.

The Nobel Prize-winning work by Roger Sperry on the polarized brain, the tripartite brain model of Paul MacLean, and the characterization of brain information storage, retrieval, and processing indicate that human will is not entirely free. There is a certain amount of unconscious drive in the lower centers and left lateral hemisphere which requires conscious control and monitoring by the higher functional areas. When the conscious control varies or is incomplete, error may result.

This implies that in work situations, like many in the lab which don't require full concentration, repetitive actions have a self-generated forward momentum, and if a worker's attention wanders, the potential for action remains. The absence of a mental double check, that is, acting before the p300 wave, can result in error. Consequently, a well-designed system, one intent on minimizing error, will accommodate this and incorporate a system of additional review to a degree proportional to the severity of negative outcome. In other words, the system can be foolproofed depending on what caliber of calamity awaits if an error occurs. This is called robustness planning and relates directly to the ability of the system design to resist uncontrolled causes of special variation.[2]

MATHEMATICAL MODELS FOR ROBUSTNESS PLANNING

David Halberstam, in his book *The Reckoning*, describes how Deming originally trained with a Bell Labs physicist, Walter A. Shewhart at a Stanford think tank with the subsequent evolution of statistical process control. Halberstam comments on Deming's remarkable work in Japan as well as Juran's powerful contributions to the early efforts in quality system design. Common to all of these gentlemen is their background in mathematical physics.

In 1963, another mathematical physicist, the originator of the term fractal, Benoit Mandelbrot, published a paper in the *IBM Journal of Research and Development* based on a fractal set known as the Cantor Dust. [3] It had to do with errors in transmission of binary information. This was the beginning of the mathematical discipline now known as chaos theory. The mathematics of chaos, and the remarkable insights provided by fractal geometry, are becoming, if not household words, at least familiar to people in many technical areas. Originally, these were mathematical curiosities used in weather prediction and coastline mapping. They are nonlinear functions, and they needed the arrival of high-speed computers to reveal their true potential.[4]

Before Mandelbrot, electrical engineers had searched for specific causes of transmission noise and for remediation by reducing the specific causes of the noise. This cause-and-effect logic is very common in Japan where it is attributed to the teachings of Confucius. It is not only common to Buddhism and Hinduism, but also to Christianity.

Statistics, however, allows inferential relationships on a probability basis. Statisticians refer to association between variables. In other words, statistical thought encourages people to think that if they do a certain thing, the probable outcome will be thus and so. Chaos theory says that there is indeed an outcome based on initial conditions, but that the outcome is completely unpredictable.

What the Cantor Dust model predicted was totally new and resulted in removing causality as an ultimate concern for electrical engineers. It predicted that a component of noise would be generated on a random basis independent of mechanical causes, that this noise level would interfere with transmission, and that no amount of fixing, fine-tuning, or otherwise cleaning up the line would ever result in an acceptably error-free transmission.

Furthermore, the noise would come in bursts following relatively long periods of quiet, but that the timing of the bursts would be unpredictable. This led to a fix quite different from the traditional approach of let's find the cause of the error and remove it.

Mandelbrot's application of the Cantor Dust model to transmission of information resulted in the installation of redundant systems for error detection. For example, the data which are sent from A to B, are then retransmitted from B to A for a second comparison. The process compares what was sent with what was received. Since the errors or dust are spread so thinly, the chance of them appearing at the same point in the forward transmission as in the backward transmission is vanishingly small.

The reason for this digression into fractal geometry is that it provides a mathematical model which may be applied to the clinical laboratory. Models clarify, and if they are truly applicable, they will also point toward solving the problem to which they have been applied. Errors in the clinical laboratory happen in a way that is similar to that described by the Cantor Dust. They happen very infrequently, and when they do, they often appear in clusters. Many times when a physician gets a wrong report, despite the lab's solemn vow never to send that physician another wrong report, the same doctor will get the next two. So what is the insight gained by knowledge of the Cantor set? It turns out that the solution is to design a system with redundancy, just as the engineers do, or to use a close cousin, foolproofing as Shigeo Shingo did. This is discussed in the following section.

CHAOS AND THE LAB

It may come as no surprise to laboratorians to find that chaos and lab management have something in common. Lab employees can run error free for a long time, and then, it always seems when it is least expected, employees become a piece of dust in the Cantor set. A specimen can be hurried into the lab, tested beautifully to within a hair of truth, mistakenly stuffed in the wrong envelope, and courier delivered in record time to the wrong doctor.

When this happens, a typical American manager embarks on a mission. The employee is rebuked, analyzed, reeducated, queried, counseled, and otherwise obliged to repent. The incident is documented and becomes a permanent part of the employee's record. When it happens again, the process is repeated. The system becomes one of iterated remediation which doesn't result in a permanent fix. It does, however, serve to heighten the stress levels of at least two individuals who are already in a high-stress environment. In short, the employee is treated to special-cause reparations for a common-cause system delivery limitation.

A Japanese manager would sit down with the employee and apologize for putting the employee in a position where he or she must take blame for a mistake. Thus the Japanese accept this component of human nature and also recognize that management has the responsibility to install systems which have suitable up-front quality measures. Thus, individuals, management, and the company do not have to suffer the embarrassment of having turned out a bad product, service, or test result.

These illustrations on the physiology of low-frequency human error demonstrate that there are only two good ways to redesign the system to prevent the error. One is by foolproofing, and the other, suggested by the Cantor set, is by redundancy. The master of foolproofing is Shigeo Shingo. Shingo apparently believes in human frailty to the extent that he recommends manufacturing procedures which can't be done wrong. For instance, to avoid stuffing a report in the wrong envelope, Shingo might recommend different size envelopes to which different reports are custom fit, or alternately, the same size envelope but color coordinated to the report—the blue report in the blue envelope.

Another advocate for recognizing and anticipating unexpected variation is Genichi Taguchi. He calls uncontrollable factors noise, and advocates accounting for these factors by robustness planning or robust system design. This planning recognizes that unexpected factors may influence system output. Thus, the best thing is to design a system which accounts for these and buffers against them. General Custer should have listened.

Redundancy is already widely used in the clinical lab. Quality control specimens on a given run are always multiple. A single control, using two standard deviation limits for acceptability, will have a one in 20, or 5-percent chance of the results falling outside these limits on a random basis (see Figure 3.6). When two controls are used, and they both fall out, the odds are only one in about 1600 that the run is acceptable, so the run is always rejected using rules for multiple control summarized by Westgard.[5]

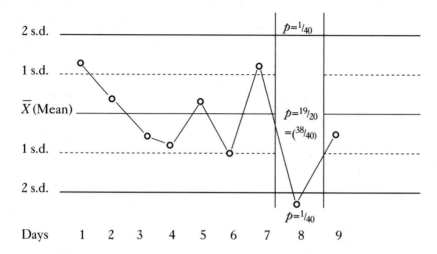

Figure 3.6: Quality control chart (Levy–Jennings plot). Quality control chart showing a point falling outside two standard deviations (s.d.) at day 8. Note that by adding up the probabilities in the vertical slice at day 8 ($^1/_{40} + ^{38}/_{40} + ^1/_{40}$), that p =1. This point must be somewhere either inside or outside the acceptance limits.

If a two-control system were used, the probability of two points falling outside the 2 s.d. limits (while the system remains in control) is the product of the individual probabilities, that is, $^1/_{40} \times ^1/_{40} = ^1/_{1600}$.

This is an example of redundancy in the mathematical sense. English majors are taught that redundancy is something superfluous, as in "exclude redundancy from spoken thought." Statisticians accept redundancy as a way to reduce error. Two controls are simply better than one. These provide much more information about the reliability of assays.

The blind control also deserves mention. With values known only to the senior tech, blind controls, when added to the run, serve as checks when used in conjunction with other control materials to release the run. The techs check their known quality values control for release of the run and the senior tech checks the blind quality control also as independent criteria for release. This redundancy removes expectational bias in addition to meeting statistical requirements.

A system with a high degree of redundancy is the hospital blood bank. Numerous double checks are in use on the floor for positive patient identification over and above the lab's efforts. Some lab systems include a repeat draw, and have the blood bank technician retest for group and type. This also illustrates redundancy compatible with the severity of downside outcome. The wrong blood can kill. This is an example of a medical procedure goal which should have a robust design. A good attitude isn't going to deliver this. Here again is a key point. None of these people want to make mistakes. Their intentions are only the best, but as Deming says, "The country is being ruined by good intentions."

Now in marketing studies, attitude and zeal are shown to correlate with increased sales. For a group of equally trained salespeople, the ones with the most energy will deliver the most goods. Even fanatic devotion on the part of lab employees, however, won't drop mistakes below a certain level, which in most clinical lab instances won't be low enough. This is, of course, anathema to traditional zero-defect managers whose philosophy is "do it right the first time." Most employees want to, but being human they simply cannot reliably deliver what is needed with the degree of reliability needed in critical case situations. They need help from the system to do this.

Many of the processes in the clinical lab already reflect this need; however, supervisor review checks, and FDA-required second signatures are frequently just that, someone signs again. If the review isn't done, this part of the redundancy cycle isn't there. Redundancy is not an easy sell. Many managers feel that redundancy tacitly encourages an individual to do slipshod work if the person feels someone will catch the mistake later.

Remember, however, that if all the traditional policies are in place for optimum employee attitude and concentration, if Mazlow's needs are satisfied, and all incentive systems are okay, the employee's best still often won't be good enough. If the system doesn't include robust design, foolproofing, or double checks, then prepare for trouble.

The Cantor Dust, neural networks, fractal geometry, transmission error, and human error all have in common naturally occurring patterns. Penrose points out that these patterns were no more invented by Mandelbrot the father of Chaos, than Schlieman, the father of modern archaeology, invented Troy. These patterns are simply there to be discovered, woven into the fabric of the universe, and as mathematicians find a way of describing them, managers find a way of applying them to work situations.

AIDS TESTING AS AN EXAMPLE OF CLINICAL REDUNDANCY

AIDS diagnosis is serious business. Any undetected carrier can spread the disease widely and quickly. So a laboratory scheme for the detection of the HIV antibody must have the highest degree of reliability. The following is an approach to meet this goal based on TQM techniques.

The degree of redundancy incorporated into the system design is relative to the severity of consequences from making a mistake and the degree of error reduction required. In the case of HIV infection diagnosis, an error can be devastating, and so labs strive to reduce error to a minimum.

In AIDS testing, one missed positive patient can be ruinous for many innocent people. For example, if the index patient, the very first HIV-positive carrier, had been identified before he had a chance to spread this new disease, the current epidemic might have been curtailed. Each positive person who is missed has the same potential for creating his or her own epidemic. The propagation is geometric.

HIV testing algorithms are based on the law of probability describing parallel redundancy. In effect this states that if one test is good, either repeating the test or doing another good test, is better. How much better can be predicted from the laws of probability. For instance, if test A is 90 percent reliable and test B is 80 percent reliable, then doing them in parallel and using both results to determine the truth would result in an overall reliability of $R = 1 - [1 - p(A)][1 - p(B)] = 1 - [1 - .9][1 - .8] = 1 - [.1][.2] = 1 - .02 = 0.98 = R$.

Thus, two systems, whose average performance is 85 percent, when used in conjunction actually perform much better than this. Converting this principle to the AIDS laboratory, the following system is derived. First an HIV–EIA screening test, which overestimates the number of people infected, is used. It is too sensitive, but this is viewed figuratively as a wide net designed to capture *all* HIV carriers. Next, a senior technologist repeats this test in duplicate after sample integrity checks. This correctly reclassifies about two-thirds of the initially positive subjects as noninfectious.

The remaining positive samples are subject to confirmatory testing. This includes several highly specific (and expensive) methods such as the western blot, recombinant assays, immunofluorescent assays, polymerase chain reactions, and culture. Each of these has associated with it a numerical probability of correct detection. In certain cases, a continued indeterminate (nondiagnostic) outcome is reviewed on an individual basis. This may call for resampling to study the donor's course over time.

In addition, this same philosophy is applied to the reagents used in the tests. Ten percent of a given lot of kits is performance checked before releasing them to the lab for general use. Further, multiple-control specimens are used at the beginning and end of a run. These controls mimic human serum or plasma. Additional controls are blind, their status known only to a senior technologist who will release a run only on 100-percent accurate reporting of all controls. Further, instrument performance checks must be within preestablished limits.

Increasingly, senior personnel review potentially reactive results and check them for any discrepancies along the way. The final report of a confirmed positive result is evaluated by supervisory personnel on its way to final review and release.

In this way, a degree of redundancy sufficient to assure maximum reliability of this highly critical operation is used. The system catches errors before a critical situation can occur.

Colonel James Damato, Ph.D., of the U.S. Army, has published an example of the extent necessary to apply this paradigm to the practice of testing for the HIV antibody. He estimates a false positive rate of one in a million.[6] This is within the six-sigma goal so often used in U.S. industry as a target of excellence. Six sigma is actually a maximum error rate of 3.4 per million.

In conclusion, the degree of reliability of a health care system must be balanced in terms of cost and benefit. Quality costs are a well-understood facet of the teachings of Juran and Deming. Caution, however, should be used in applying traditional cost-benefit analysis to a virus like HIV that strikes through the reproductive route. Too little recognition of the harsh consequences of indifference could be an invitation to join other species which became extinct for reasons far less obvious.

REDUNDANCY AND CLINICAL SIGNIFICANCE

In 1985 the National Heart Lung and Blood Institute of the National Institutes of Health (NIH) began the National Cholesterol Education Program (NCEP). This program was modeled after a similar earlier program which had been designed to alert Americans that high blood pressure was the silent killer. This program was the first such NIH program to inform the entire U.S. population that elevated blood pressure was a risk factor and to establish guidelines for what pressures represented risk and what sort of treatment regimens were recommended.

The NCEP had established two committees when I joined the program. These were the Adult Treatment Panel, composed mostly of physicians, and the Lab Standardization Panel, on which I served. The purpose of the standardization panel was to study the error components of cholesterol assays and to recommend ways to minimize these variables and to achieve a degree of standardization with regard to this assay countrywide.[7]

Even for a routine clinical assay such as cholesterol, the panel recognized error components relating both to lab testing and to the preanalytical phase of testing. Although both of these are small, as an aggregate, they can be sufficiently large to improperly classify the subject with regard to risk.

Since a high cholesterol can result in the subject being put on expensive long-term therapy for the condition, the panel recognized that to guarantee correct classification one needed multiple assays on multiple samples. In addition, these assays had to be done on a system which was referenced to a standard material traceable to the National Institute of Standards and Technology method and the CDC-reference cholesterol standards. Since CLIA '88 specifies that assay methods now be validated, chapter 6 and Appendix B detail the statistics and error analysis of similar methods. For now, there are two major qualitative considerations which I would like to emphasize.

First, it was a fascinating experience to observe a national program unfold. Initial surveys indicated that virtually none of the American public, and only a small percentage of the physician population, were aware that cholesterol was a cardiovascular risk factor. Further, the physicians were largely using outdated and even dangerous treatment methods when they were treating high cholesterol at all.

When the program ended, most Americans knew that diet and exercise were important and had largely bought into the program. The issue of cholesterol almost became lost in the larger awareness of how to achieve a healthy life-style. There was actually a bigger payoff than the original effort had foreseen.

Secondly, the standardization panel was striving for an analytical error component of 5 percent coefficient of variation (CV). The panel estimated that this could be reached by doing duplicate analyses on four separate patient specimens. From a practical standpoint, the panel finally recommended that at least two measurements on separate occasions be done prior to making any medical decision based on these results.

Individuals with high cholesterol are no danger to anyone but themselves. A person with the human immunodeficiency virus can be a potential epidemic.

Redundancy is applied then in keeping with clinical significance. It is widely accepted that a blood sugar level of ± 5 percent is adequate to permit the physician to correctly classify subjects with glucose abnormalities. Increasing the accuracy of the measurement would simply increase cost without derived benefit.

Similarly, the NCEP arrived at a long-range cholesterol target of ±3 percent CV, in order to permit a similarly correct classification. In AIDS testing, however, techniques to approach the theoretical limit of reliability are employed.

NOTES

1. D. Joe Boone, Ph.D., "Literature Review of Research Related to the Clinical Laboratory Improvement Amendments of 1988," *Archives of Pathology and Laboratory Medicine* 116 (1992): 681.

2. Ronald D. Snee, "Creating Robust Work Processes," *Quality Progress* 26 (February 1993): 37–41.

3. Benoit Mandelbrot, "A New Model for the Clustering of Error in Telephone Circuits," *IBM Journal of Research and Development* 7 (1963): 224–236.

4. Benoit Mandelbrot, *The Fractal Geometry of Nature* (New York: W. H. Freeman & Co., 1983), 79–82.

5. James O. Westgard and T. Groth, "A Predictive Value Model for Quality Control: Effects of the Prevalence of Errors on the Performance of Control Procedures," *American Journal of Clinical Pathology* 80 (1983): 49–56. For early documented use of SPC in the clinical lab, see James O. Westgard et al., "A Multi-Rule Shewhart Chart for Quality Control in Clinical Chemistry," *Clinical Chemistry* 27 (1981): 493–501.

6. James J. Damato, Ph.D. et al., "Resolution of Indeterminate HIV-1 Test Data Using Department of Defense HIV-1 Testing Program," *Laboratory Medicine* 22, no. 2 (February 1991): 107–113.

7. Herbert K. Naito, "Current Status of Blood Cholesterol Measurement in Clinical Laboratories in the United States: A Report from the Laboratory Standardization Panel of the National Cholesterol Education Program," *Clinical Chemistry* 34 (1988): 193.

SUGGESTED READING

Bloom, Floyd E., and Arlyne Lazerson. *Brain, Mind and Behavior*. New York: W. H. Freeman, 1988.

Davies, Paul. *The Cosmic Blueprint*. New York: Orion Productions, 1988.

Gleick, James. *Chaos—Making a New Science*. New York: Penguin Books, 1988.

Heller, Wendy. "Of One Mind—Second Thoughts About the Brain's Dual Nature." *The Sciences* (May/June 1990): 38–44.

Penrose, Roger. *The Emperor's New Mind*. New York: W. H. Freeman, 1990.

Restak, Richard M. *The Brain, The Last Frontier*. Garden City, New York: Doubleday, 1979.

Rosenfeld, Anne H. *Archaeology of Affect*. Washington, D.C.: National Institute of Mental Health and National Institutes of Health, 1976.

Shimbun, Nikkan. *Poka-Yoke*. Red Bluff, Calif.: QCI International, 1989.

Sperry, Roger W. "Lateral Specialization of Cerebral Function in Surgically Separated Hemispheres." In *The Psychophysiology of Thinking*, edited by F. J. McGuigan, and R. A. Schoonover. New York: Academic Press, 1973.

4

The Tools of TQM

The basic TQM tools are provided by way of introduction. They are basic to the quality effort, and although they predate TQC, the quality effort will not proceed smoothly without an understanding of their contribution to the movement.

MEETINGS

It is essential to know how to run a meeting well. There are only a few key things which must be done to assure this. In her book *Deming Management at Work*, Mary Walton relates how the Hospital Corporation of America adopted TQM partially in response to a poll of managers which indicated that they felt they were wasting most of their time in meetings. This is a hazard in companies that encourage meetings to handle any problem or opportunity, irrespective of how trivial.

When deploying TQM there may be a tendency to have process improvement groups which address overly mundane matters. As a result, it is necessary to have some sort of control over the matters these groups review without restraining the creative juices that flow from unbridled enthusiasm that accompanies an unrestrained format. Still, meetings can become part of the problem rather than part of the solution if they are not run well.

99

The key points in a meeting start with the timely arrival of all participants. Usually the facilitator or chair will be late as this is a routine way of showing power. This type of leader should be shut out and a designated backup should take over. Have a phone in the meeting room and have someone take "late" excuses, which the group may or may not want to acknowledge. Unplug the phone 10 minutes after the meeting is scheduled to start.

Having arrived at a timely beginning, the chair should be designated and the meeting run by parliamentary procedure. This means the chair must recognize attendees prior to them speaking. This must be skillfully done by the chair in order to allow for extemporizing, but at the same time, the chair must dissuade monopoly of the floor by the inevitable vocal personalities. Parliamentary procedure, though, gives the chair the power to regulate the meeting and to make it expeditious.

The chair and the facilitator should be separate. The facilitator's job is to make sure that the tools are correctly used and that standard operating procedure is followed. The chair keeps the meeting on track and runs it efficiently.

This is the format for a good-sized, formal, scheduled meeting. There are many opportunities in the deployment of TQM in which smaller ad hoc groups will be meeting. Thus, a variation of the outlined procedure will be needed. The primary difference in the small group meeting is that there may be no chairperson, simply a facilitator. In this case, this person assumes a dual role, deals with the organization less formally, and takes on the role of recalling the group to task if it strays too far from the point.

A meeting agenda is a must. Even if it is only a few lines, or even one line, the meeting must have a purpose, and an agenda is the first step toward organizing the group by focusing attention on the items for review. An agenda also serves as a record of who was invited to review what, when, and where. Most important, though, the agenda tells why the meeting was held in the first place. The meeting goals should be part of the agenda. This helps to keep the meeting focused.

A recorder should be part of the meeting if warranted. Even if not, the meeting should be summarized briefly and sent to a central point for incorporation into the company's quality records. The record then becomes a historical report of the deliberations and a learning tool for others who may later address similar situations.

The meeting should end on an upward note. Some call this a path forward. It can happen that the meeting didn't go especially well in that not as much was accomplished as expected. Rather than end here, identify a positive note and a way to follow up in a positive way. The chair should adjourn on time. This sounds simple, but meetings that drag are not only inefficient, but they also play havoc with attendees' schedules which were contingent on the meeting stopping when the meeting notice said it would stop.

THE FIVE W's AND ONE H

The primary tenets of journalistic reporting, who, what, why, when, where, and how, are an example of TQC tools that come from other areas of specialization and have been successfully woven into the web of TQM.

In many cases of applying either the management or the QC tools, certain questions about various line items are asked to assure completeness of the analysis. For instance, the Japanese suggest, ask why five times. George Nakamura of Scripps Institute says, "The man who knows *how* will always have a job. The man who knows *why* will always be his boss."

Of the five W's and one H—who, what, why, when, where, and how—why is the most important. In many cases, it is also the most difficult to answer.

As an example, take the simple acquisition of a new instrument. Who will run it, when will it arrive, where shall it go, what manufacturer will be selected, and how will it be installed? These are all questions that must be answered before routine testing on the machine can begin. The why question is generally asked prior to any of the others, and it is frequently asked by accounting for purposes of cost justification. If the reasons don't make good sense, competitive forces may result in diversion of the cash elsewhere.

If accounting asks the question, then the only good answers relate to money—how much is saved or how much more may be generated from the acquisition. Using the quality expectations attendant to the purchase shouldn't be overlooked in fleshing out a response. This would include aspects drawn from a 6-M Ishikawa diagram, that is, men, machine, materials, methods, measurement, and milieu. Justification would then include the following:

- *Men:* The same quality or better quality results could be achieved using fewer operators and/or less-skilled operators. The new process will free trained people for more productive work.
- *Machine:* It could add quality factors such as positive patient identification, computer interfacial capability, less sample needed, and faster throughput.

- *Measurement:* More, different, or new analyses could be achieved. Similarly, better accuracy, precision, and/or reliability could be accomplished.
- *Materials:* Less sample or reagent may be needed, and a better preventive maintenance program that is cheaper and more accessible could be used.
- *Methods:* Any or all of the following could be achieved: new or updated technology; more acceptable or readable output (for example, reporting through the computer); and automatic quality control graph capability which saves tech time and automates the quality process.
- *Milieu:* Advantages include reduced space, less noise and heat, and easier reagent change capability. Reagents could be stored in a more compact way. Thus, less lab disorder is associated with servicing and maintaining the instrument.

This little exercise shows the use of the 5 W's and one H. It combines them with an Ishikawa diagram for the justification as well as the implementation of a new equipment purchase.

THE GANTT CHART

The Gantt chart is used as an additional tool for effecting the process startup and charting the project course with time. As a minimum, the Gantt should have answers to the 5W–1H questions. Stratification, or further breakdown, should be used too. This means, for instance, that there may be many how questions: How to order, how to pay, how to train, how to schedule personnel, and so forth.

The Gantt chart, named after Henry L. Gantt in 1917, is used for project scheduling. It is another very basic organizational tool. It is widely used because it is so easy to understand and so practical.

The typical Gantt chart plots action items versus time in a sequential way. It starts with the first items in a project and arranges subsequent actions in a progressive way, showing which items need to be completed before others can begin, and which items can proceed in parallel or independently.

The Gantt chart has been criticized because of its inability to show interaction between steps in a more complex operation. For instance, in 1950 the scheduling of the *Polaris* submarine assembly used the program evaluation and review technique (PERT) which allows for more advanced insights, such as determination of critical path. Although the Navy makes some very complicated things, the principle behind assembling the submarine was to make sure the engines were in before the hull was closed.

This may sound trivial, but on the local level moving a blood bank refrigerator uses the same principles. If no one has considered whether the refrigerator will fit through the door, then the last step in the process may be dropping the fridge in through the roof by crane.

The Gantt charting process has added some improvements such as resource allocation and parallel expense tracking. Also, newly available computer software makes organizing and redoing a Gantt easier than in the past. The Gantt is a big help in visualizing a project. Figure 4.1 shows a Gantt chart of a typical lab activity.

THE SEVEN QUALITY CONTROL TOOLS

In Japan, the number seven has a special significance as it has throughout history and even prehistory. The sacred character of the number is thought to be derived from the lunar week. The prehistorian Alexander Marschak reports seeing the figure inscribed on bones 30,000 years old, and seven dots appear repeatedly on the walls of the cave inhabited 17,000 years ago at Lascaux.

The Japanese refer to the seven QC tools and the seven new tools or management tools. This Japanese emphasis on the number seven gives westerners the impression that either all the tools have the same importance or that they are always used in sets of seven when problem solving or planning management strategy. This is like saying that all 88 keys on the piano have the same value or are meant to be played simultaneously. The use of these tools is an art, and this skill can be developed just like that of a concert pianist.

In effect, these are but two groups of devices which have broad applicability. The management tools help in decision making consistent with hoshin kanri, or management by policy. The QC tools help to analyze error, in particular the error of special causes or assignable error, so that the system reduces to an in-control process which can then be handled in conventional fashion. The process is then amenable to process improvement or kaizen, in which the QC tools again play a key role.

The seven QC tools are

1. Flowchart
2. Ishikawa, cause-and-effect, or fishbone diagram
3. Check sheet

Subject: Courier addition
Object: To have a trained pickup and delivery driver ready with all equipment in a two-week period.

Feb

Activity	Resource	Cost ($)	1	2	3	4	5	6	7	8	9	10	11	12	13	14	15
Order car	Transportation	400/mo	X														
Take delivery on car	Pool	100			X												
Customize car (racks, company logo)	Transportation	500				X---X---X---X---X											
Deliver car to pool	Transportation	10							X								
Identify candidate	Personnel	100	X---X														
Train in pickup	Education	300			X---X---X												
Train in delivery	Education	300					X---X---X									
Train in SOPs	Education	300									X---X---X					
Train on the job	Transportation	400												X---X---X---X		
Certify and release to job	Transportation/ education/ personnel/	200															X

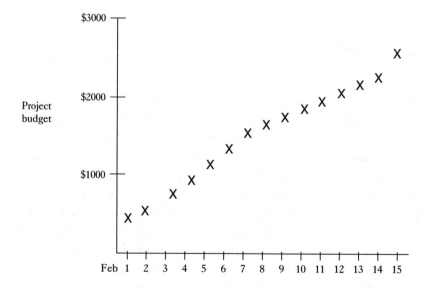

Figure 4.1: Gantt chart—lab process scheduling.

4. Histogram and Pareto diagram
5. Run chart/control chart
6. Scatter diagram
7. Stratification

In addition, there are four advanced tools. These are

1. Design of experiments
2. Taguchi analysis
3. Multivariate analysis
4. Regression analysis

Sometimes the QC tools can be viewed as a formal way to address and solve problems. At a seminar in which managers addressed problem-solving types of management, they said that a management style geared to problem solving will eventually effect an equilibrium state in which each series of problems solved will result in an equal number of new problems to solve. This is the familiar stamping-out-fires management style. This type of management never focuses long enough on the overall system, but instead sees only the short-term symptoms of the overall system problem.

Even in a medical sense, treating symptoms is only acceptable if the disease is self-limiting. In a business situation, system problems rarely cure themselves, and so symptomatic treatment is a never-ending process. This, however, keeps many managers busy and satisfied that they are contributing something, and indeed they are. They are maintaining mediocrity.

These tools should be viewed not so much as problem-solving methods, but more as ways to close the gap between where the process is now and where it should be. The distance between the status quo and the targeted process performance is the opportunity for improvement. Now examine the process improvement techniques and some of the tools used to make improvement happen.

Flowchart

A flowchart is a tool used to visualize a process so that the steps in the process can be clearly seen. Flowcharting should be used in all lab processes as a matter of course. Behind each and every lab procedure should be the flowchart representing the process. At any time in which the procedure comes under review, the flowchart should be the first step in the analysis of the process and its projected improvement.

Flowcharting is the procedural equivalent of graphing data. Ungraphed data are very difficult to visualize, but graphing clearly shows relationships. Similarly, a flowchart presents the mind with a clear view of a process from beginning to end.

Flowcharts have symbols which are standardized by the American National Standards Institute (ANSI). These are the football-shaped symbols indicating start or stop; the rectangle for the process step or component; the parallelogram for the action step (many use the rectangle for this as well); and the diamond for the decision (yes/no) step.

In addition, modern flowcharts have some ad hoc symbols which have obvious meanings. There are computer programs available to help in flowcharting. These are strongly recommended because they let the user choose the standard symbols, in addition to providing some of the newer symbols, and they automatically center the words in the process blocks.

Flowcharting, then, is a tool which can be used in both planning and diagnosis. In the planning phase, the flowchart is the quality tool analogue of management tools such as the Gantt and PERT charts. These give a holistic view of the steps of a project dimensioned against time, whereas the flowchart gives an overall view of an ongoing process. Time isn't a factor in the flowchart. The flowchart looks the same whether the process goes fast or slow.

The flowchart can also be used to position *control stations*. This is a term used by Juran, which in the lab situation is equivalent to in-process quality reviews. In the manufacturing sense, control stations are based near work stations and are responsible for sampling a station's output prior to passing it on for further manufacturing use.

In the lab sense, the flowchart shows that, at a particular point, a quality control check is required. This need not be done by a separate person or group; in fact, the modern trend is to have the in-process QC work done by the individuals responsible for the work. If at all possible—and in the lab this is not always the case—review is most effective when done by other individuals.

For example, in the setup of a batch processing analyzer, an early quality check would be to verify the specimen tubes against the work list. This is most often done by the operator, after an initial check done perhaps by accessioning. There must be positive identification that the specimen going into the machine for analysis belongs to the patient so identified. Whether this is a bar code scan or a visual scan, it is a necessary QC check, and the flowchart should clearly delineate the necessity of this stage.

There is also an integrated flowchart which integrates function with responsible department, supervisory group, or individual. The groupings are arrayed across the top of the page and the flowchart proceeds down the page, but each functional step appears under the appropriate header indicating the who behind the what. Figure 4.2 is a flowchart showing the laboratory role in patient diagnosis.

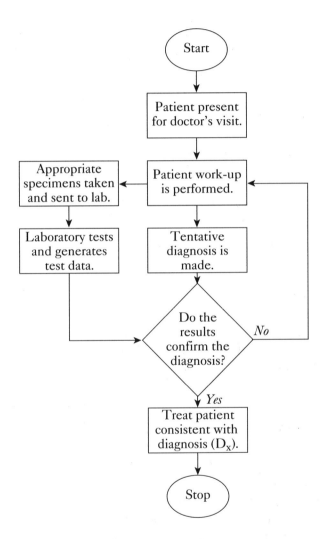

Figure 4.2: Flowchart of the laboratory role in patient diagnosis. The start and stop blocks are easily seen. The process steps use the rectangular block, and the decision block is the diamond shape. Usually a flowchart will be designed so that each process block has only a single input and output; however, if the subject is easily understood, parallel processes can be accommodated without confusion. An example of an integrated flowchart is Figure 3.1 (p. 72). There, each department responsible for the action shows the process occurring under its own heading. This integrates the what with the who.

The Ishikawa Diagram, Fishbone, or Cause-and-Effect Diagram

Having analyzed the process by flowcharting, the next step to assess the causes of system variation is usually the Ishikawa diagram. The idea is to visually depict the separate aspects of the process. To help include the important ones, the 6-M diagram is used. This is simply a mnemonic to help remind the user of the six major ribs attaching to the vertebrae of the fishbone.

These vertebrae are men, machine, materials, methods, measurement, and milieu, or as commonly seen but more difficult to remember, personnel, equipment, materials, methods, measurement, and environment. Regardless of how these ribs are remembered, start with these six bones as a minimum. They are considered the components of a process. Outline the diagram as in Figure 4.3 and add subprocesses to the six major ribs. Any reasonable technique (for instance brainstorming), can be used to identify as many component processes as possible. At this point prioritizing these is not the issue, but identifying and visually representing them are important.

Identification of the component processes includes the following:

- *Men:* These are the people contributing to the process. Important aspects are their training and education levels needed for process performance. Licensing or other regulatory concerns and other physical or intellectual preferences are applicable to the process.
- *Machine:* This relates to the equipment used in the processes with regard to its characteristics and how it is applied to the analytical method. Quality factors to be considered may be positive patient identification, computer interfacial capability, sampling capabilities, and throughput. The equipment is frequently judged from a productivity standpoint, that is, how much output per unit time or per dollar reagent cost.
- *Measurement:* The separation of measurement from machine can be better appreciated by referring to a manufacturing analogue. In a metal fabrication assembly line, the machines can be stampers, cutters, grinders, and other metalworking machines. The measurement is the QC measurement which allows the assembly to pass a given point. These tools are frequently gages, micrometers, and calipers which are subject to wear. In the lab, the measurement and the machine are frequently the same, but the quality of the analytical outcome is dependent on a well-maintained instrument.

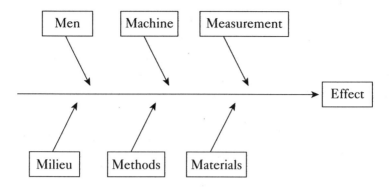

Figure 4.3: Ishikawa, cause-and-effect, or fishbone diagram. The 6-M cause-and-effect diagram relates six common causes to system variability.

- *Materials*: Materials usage refers to hardware, sampling cups, chart paper, reagent use, and associated preventive maintenance.
- *Methods:* This relates to the analytical technology which, in turn, may generate a convenient information output, storage and retrieval, or an assay incorporating nonspecific interferences.
- *Milieu:* Environmental concerns center around the space taken up by the machine and extend as far as the noise or smell it makes while operating. The interaction of the machine with the environment in terms of reagent storage and change are important as well.

A digression on the particular emphasis on the visual character of the tools may be helpful at this point. Chapter 2, on the theory of profound knowledge, discusses the fact that brain researchers are now using a convention of a right brain/left brain bipolar description of the way the brain processes information. They divide the brain into two broad functional areas. In most people, the left side deals with speech and quantitative functions. It is the vocal side and handles written and spoken information and appears to process data in a sequential, numerical, and analytical way.

The right brain, on the other hand, is the artistic side and deals with data in a more abstract fashion. In addition, it is also the creative side of the brain, although by itself, it is nonverbal. Understanding this allows humans to understand the need for pictures. The improvements resulting from a visually presented process may have a more original and creative character than the same process presented in narrative or tabular form.

Check Sheets

In proceeding from the Ishikawa diagram to Pareto analysis it becomes necessary to collect data in an organized fashion for use in assigning prime causes of system variability. This is the 80/20 rule of Pareto. But to get to the Pareto histograms, it is necessary to collect data based on the causes generated in the fishbone. A carefully designed check sheet can help.

The check sheet should have on it all parameters that the customer views as important. The check sheet should be usable in the line operation with little training, and it should allow line people to collect data for later analysis by various methods. In a production sense, if a good product is one with a shiny finish, then the number and location of dull finishes or finishes with dents, scratches, knocks, rust spots, and so forth will be counted and recorded on the check sheet.

In a service sense, the number of times that turnaround time (TAT) exceeds 24 hours (or the optimal TAT) is recorded for a given department. The check sheet may include type of test, shift, individual, and enough selected components of the process to determine potential causes of special variation. If all these things are lumped together the smoothing effect of the averaging process may obscure the special causes. Sample check sheets are shown in Appendix B.

In some cases a quantitative marker is difficult to get particularly if items of a subjective nature are under analysis. In this case, it is important to understand the differences between attributes and variables and how the tools are used with them. The tools also allow for the statistical measurement of nonquantitative operations.

One of the key elements to quantifying a process is to determine whether or not it is observable and measurable. There is a discipline of statistics which allows a quantitative estimate of a qualitative observation. This is a type of variable sampling.

In accepting a bolt for use, a template into which the bolt fits can be used. If the bolt passes (that is, it isn't a screw or nut) then it is accepted, and if not, it is rejected. If the only important function of the bolt is its diameter, which must be within a certain acceptance limit, then checking the diameter is measuring a variable. If the variable is within specs, then the unit passes into finished goods inventory.

How can something as qualitative and subjective as the pleasure of a sunset be measured? Certainly some sunsets are better than others, but the question is how much better. This relates to business practices in the many instances in which a subjective impression needs quantification. The food industry is very good at this because it needs to market things which have visual appeal, nice smell, right feel, and good taste. None of these is easily quantified, but a great deal of time and money can be wasted launching a new product meant to please four of the five senses but doesn't.

The sunset which simply has visual appeal can be dissected further. The visual allure can be broken down into subsets of color, clouds, duration, afterglow, and so on. This can be scaled to reduce the subjective attributes to a quantitative scale of variables. This can be analyzed by statistics of discontinuous distributions to tell whether last night's sunset was statistically different from tonight's sunset. Cosmetics designers use the same techniques.

So in designing the check sheet, don't hesitate to use both qualitative and quantitative aspects of the service or production component. Use both attributes and variables. Statistics can handle either, and Pareto analysis is amenable to both.

Pareto Analysis

Named after the Italian count who developed it, Pareto analysis follows naturally from the fishbone diagram in that data suggest that 80 percent of the system variation follows from 20 percent of the causes. Sometimes referred to as the 80/20 rule, this acknowledgment allows managers to initially focus on a relatively small number of sources of process variation, while expecting a much greater reduction in process variability.

The Pareto diagram is presented as a histogram with the most predominant cause of process variation to the far left. It is important to recognize that the Pareto diagram should be based on actual measurement. The speculation phase has ended with the fishbone diagram, and the purpose of the Pareto analysis is to find the longest bone or two. While the prioritization can be done by continued speculation, the longer bones are best based on measured parameters. If possible, a quality characteristic must be derived so that this process capability parameter can be plotted over time. In this fashion, visual evidence is displayed to indicate process improvement. See Figure 4.4 for a Pareto diagram.

Run Diagrams and Control Diagrams

A run diagram is a chart of a quality parameter over time. The idea of the PDCA process is to generate process improvement. This is difficult to prove without a measurable parameter which can be viewed over time. There has been more than one instance in which the process was made worse due to wrong initial work-up. This, however, is the beauty of the

Deming process and the PDCA cycle; that is, tacit or implicit check mechanisms are placed to monitor change, whether or not the change results in improvement.

The run diagram is used to monitor progress. Its use is limited to graphically depicting the change (hopefully reflecting progress) that the new procedures have wrought. Its use is as a short-term indicator. The control diagrams can be run diagrams with limits set from statistical analysis of the data used to generate the run diagram. These are like the Levy–Jennings control charts used in the clinical lab. On the other hand, the control chart, in traditional TQM usage, is used only to study the process variability under the new set of conditions, and the control limits are used to determine if the new process is in control. After this the control chart is discontinued and other surveillance means are used to assure that the process continues in control. In the clinical lab, however, the most

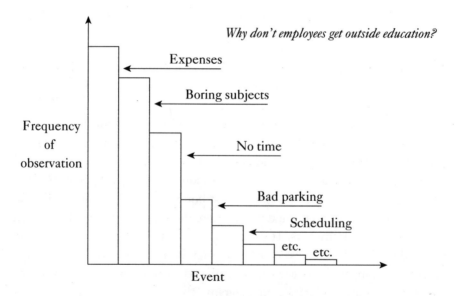

Figure 4.4: Pareto diagram. Named after Vilfredo Pareto who pointed out that most of the money was in the hands of the privileged few, this principle was applied to process analysis by Joseph Juran. In the example, no time and scheduling may be related and should be added to establish a different priority. The components of the Pareto diagram should be independent. In this way, a business can allocate finite resources in the most expeditious manner. The Pareto diagram focuses these finite company resources in the highest priority areas, those in which process improvement will have the greatest effect.

appropriate use of the run diagram would be to track change, followed by determination of statistically derived limits and conversion over to a control diagram.

In summary, a run diagram is a visual representation of the performance of the system with time. Inspection tells whether the system delivery has improved, worsened, or remained relatively constant.

The control chart is a plot of system performance with time in which upper and lower control limits have been placed to guide the user in qualifying production to a set standard. The limits can be derived statistically, or they can be based on other criteria indicating good performance such as user-defined acceptability limits. The conventional lab example is the widely used Levy–Jennings plots with statistically set limits and acceptability criteria based on the use of multiple controls. Control diagrams are more thoroughly examined in chapter 6.

Scatter Diagrams and Regression Analysis

This is an example of repackaging Japanese TQC for American use and in de-emphasizing their culturally derived fixation with the number seven. Remember that the seven QC tools might imply that the tools are equally important and have equally broad utility, but, in fact, this isn't true. In addition, the advanced QC concepts may, in fact, be more routinely used and have broader purpose than some of the original seven. This is particularly true in an institution where the statistical help is a mature service and readily available to operating groups.

Scatter diagrams are a case in point. They have a limited use in relating cause and effect between two entities. The simplest example is plotting height against weight of a population and finding that, although there is considerable scatter, a 6' 5" NFL lineman is quite a bit heavier than a 4' 7" gymnast. The scatter comes from the fact that not all people 6' 5" are in the NFL and weigh 320 pounds. Some tall people are thin, and some short people are not.

In implying causality from a scatter diagram, inspection is used first, but one of the advanced QC techniques, regression analysis, is used to determine the reliability of the inferences drawn from plotting two parameters on a sheet of graph paper. Just the fact that they are both on the same sheet of paper yields a correlation of sorts. Whether they are related through cause and effect can be clarified using regression analysis. This is a good example of viewing the world through the eyes of a statistician, since true causality cannot be proven but only inferred using statistical techniques like this.

As an example, the scatter diagram might be used to determine if the right bones have been chosen in the Ishikawa diagram. In using the diagram, causality is inferred, but at some point in the problem analysis, the causes are going to have to be determined for real and quantified. If this is not done then the problem analysis is based on speculation. While the results can be quite good using the check functions of the PDCA cycle, there are cases in which trial and error is simply not an option, and in these cases the analysis of cause must be done with great care and thoroughness.

Another way of looking at these tools is under the broader heading of correlation analysis. This technique may be thought of as proceeding in stages as follows: (1) scatter diagram, (2) curve fitting, (3) regression analysis, and (4) correlation coefficient calculation. It is one way of comparing things, and it is examined in more detail in chapter 6.

Stratification

This is the easiest of the tools to understand. Deming says that in Japan the boundaries of the system are the boundaries of the country. Japan is a system using raw materials, people, and money to make products, goods, and services. The tools, in theory, can be used to analyze special- and common-cause variation within that system. In a practical sense, they are used to study subsystems and processes within the countrywide system.

Stratification is the process whereby the same tools are used to analyze subsystems in an increasingly meticulous manner. Businesses within the country are split into categories, the categories into individual business functions, and then into single businesses. The operations within the single business are appraised in this way until the bones in the Ishikawa diagram are detached and subjected to check sheet, Pareto, and run/control diagrams. Whenever a problem appears somewhat intractable because of its size, stratification should be considered as a way to make it easy to handle.

The Advanced QC Tools

The advanced QC tools are regression analysis, design of experiments, Taguchi analysis, and multivariate analysis. These techniques are used, frequently in combination, to assess the effects of individual components of multicomponent systems on the system output. This is done experimentally, and the data are analyzed statistically.

For example, one of the monomer plants of a major oil company was analyzed to determine why it was falling down. There was corrosion, and after too short a time, pipes sprung leaks. The conventional remedy would be to smooth out some of the right angles in the plumbing, to change the metal the pipe was made from, and to insert some sacrificial electrodes. These electrodes are designed to undergo electrolytic corrosion preferentially to the pipe. If the wrong material is used, however, the pipe will corrode first, protecting the sacrificial electrode, which is not the idea at all. This is sort of like a bulb burning out to protect a fuse.

The company used two methods to analyze this problem: design of experiments and multivariate analysis. Note that Taguchi analysis is a variant of design of experiments.

The plant flow stream had seven chemical components flowing through it, and their concentrations varied from zero to very high levels. The flow rates varied from slow and laminar to fast and turbulent. In addition, the piping available was three grades of stainless steel and two grades of carbon steel. Further, there were a variety of sacrificial electrodes from which to choose. The problem, then, was to select the correct piping material for various points in the existing miles of piping to match the chemical makeup and speed of the flow stream and to add in a choice sacrificial electrode if this would help things.

The design of experiments application used five types of steel, several flow rates, and different chemical makeups of the plant stream. This was done in the lab over a week. The data reduction and matrix data analysis took longer and eventually resulted in a plant redesign consistent with integrating the plumbing and storage materials to their flow streams.

The point of all this is to illustrate the complexity of these procedures and the complexity of the processes which the procedures can address. Note that both the design and the data analysis are not for the uninitiated. Experimental design in itself is fraught with pitfalls into which quite experienced people have fallen. There are new methods for experimental design which are currently being debated. These methods work best when done in conjunction with a technical support department which has the expertise and computer support needed to make these techniques work. Without this, these methods are not only more trouble than they are worth, but they are also more likely to mislead. In conclusion then, by all means use these advanced tools if the resources are available and the problem is sufficiently complex to warrant it. An example of lab use of design of experiments is shown in chapter 6.

THE SEVEN MANAGEMENT TOOLS

The QC tools in conjunction with the PDCA cycle can be used to support the concept of kaizen. They can be used to inaugurate the process of gradual and continual improvement. These tools are designed to identify opportunities or problems in a system or process, to prioritize, sort, and quantitate those problems, and to reduce or eliminate the main causes of special variation in the process. In this way, the gap between current system delivery and projected or desired system performance is narrowed or closed.

Recently, the Japanese refer to the seven new tools, which are directed at predicting system shortcomings before they cause problems. In this sense, they are used in the planning phase of the Deming cycle. These seven tools are

1. Affinity diagram
2. Relationship diagram
3. Process decision program chart (PDPC) analysis
4. Matrix diagram
5. Matrix data analysis
6. Systematic diagram
7. Arrow diagrams

As a simple point of clarification, all of the QC tools, all of the new tools, the four advanced tools, and SPC were first developed in the United States. The Japanese then added kaizen, hoshin kanri, and quality function deployment.

Affinity Diagram

Brainstorming is frequently used and generally well understood. The chairperson goes around the meeting room asking each person, in turn, to reflect on the subject under review. The thoughts are recorded. This continues until it becomes obvious that nothing more of note can be generated. Often a rating system is applied in which the group prioritizes the suggestions.

A way of formalizing this process is the affinity diagram. Here, thoughts on the subject are written down on 3" × 5" self-adhesive papers (for example, Post-it™ notes). This may be done prior to the meeting if the subject is known well in advance. Otherwise the spontaneous generation of these ideas in the meeting is the accepted way. All parties should be allowed to contribute. Since the offerings are silently written down, there is no domination by the most vocal members. Everyone has a say.

The group then arranges the ideas such that thoughts share a certain affinity. This is again done silently to avoid a vocal bias. This may be an equilibrium process with certain contributions being shifted from pile to pile but eventually a reasonable number of affinity areas will emerge, and the group can then recapitulate the thought of each area into a cogent statement that the group can then use for further work. A number of related piles will result. A small miscellaneous pile may also occur.

Alternatively, the group may be lucky enough that a card in each batch will represent the essence of that batch without requiring a rewrite. Affinity diagrams are generally used for large conceptual types of problems which are difficult to handle in a well-organized way by other means. Affinity diagrams are not especially useful for less complicated problems in which a quick brainstorming can focus quickly on the right aspects for later review. Affinity diagrams, then, should be used for speculation and definition of broadly based problems.

In the discussion on the Ishikawa diagram, it was suggested that the 6-M components of a system be used as starting points for analysis. Certainly other systems have different components, but the 6-M are basic and will lead to good things.

The Ishikawa diagram can also be used as a means-and-objective diagram where the backbone points to the objective and the ribs are means. When using this diagram for means/objective analysis, Gitlow suggests using the outcome of the affinity diagram as the ribs. If the brainstorming process yields a reasonable number of major categories, then these can be used as the major means generating the outcome. In addition, the piles under the major headings can be used as the lesser ribs. In this way a very tight focus is maintained on the process analysis, and it flows naturally from the group input. Using a 6-M approach in this instance, where the means are predefined, frequently results in the group generating some rather abstract and occasionally pointless input simply because the rib calls for it. In a similar fashion, the output from an affinity diagram can be used to generate the relationship diagram.

Relationship Diagram

The relationship diagram is another way to study a very complex problem. From the diagram, the root causes and root effects become clear. The relationship diagram is used in the planning stages, and one way of getting the relationships for the diagram is the output of the organized brainstorming from the affinity diagram. The affinity groups are arranged in a pattern such that the relationship is determined among the groups.

Whereas in the affinity diagram the affinities are grouped and arranged for discussion, the relationship diagram ties these together with arrows which point from cause to effect. If there are missing parts, then more brainstorming is usually used to fill in the gaps. In this way a pictorial diagram emerges which relates component causes with potential effects, with the whole of the complex process undergoing review.

The root cause is the circumstance on which the team must focus its efforts to affect process change. Secondary root effects also result from the relationship diagram. These are red herrings. They result from the root cause, and the traditional mistake is to direct remedial efforts at rectifying the red herrings. This is a waste of time because the root cause which generated them in the first place will remain intact.

Process Decision Program Chart

A PDPC is generated from processes which identify opportunities for improvement in the overall process either before or after the process is implemented. The chart results from a combination of earlier techniques known as failure mode and effect analysis (FMEA), design review, and fault-tree analysis (FTA).

The overall focus of these techniques is to shift attention away from the strictly front-end planning function and design of the process, to a far-reaching spotlight which centers on what-if effects (contingency planning). The questions on which these techniques center relate to predicting what may go awry with the process at various points and predict the seriousness of the malfunction, and implement contingency plans if these things happen.

Design review is a technique where the final process design is reviewed by someone other than the planners themselves. The idea behind this is that even though experts in TQM designed the process, a different perspective may spot problems in the design which may develop with time. To effectively use design review, the following criteria must be met.

- The review must be formal, scheduled, and to set criteria.
- The review must be done by system experts other than designers.

The criteria for the review are generally those set by the customer or end user of the process. An agenda for the meeting is set, and the process is reviewed for overall suitability which includes both immediate user suitability as well as potential long-term suitability. The review committee needs sufficient time to digest the process and review any other information associated with it. The agendas are circulated prior to the meetings, minutes of the meeting are kept, and recommendations for change and improvement are generated as a meeting summary. The purpose of the design review committee is to remove any developing monopoly that may occur when process improvement groups become too inbred.

Methods the design review committee may use are FTA and FMEA. These two processes have a mirror-image relationship. Both are meant to detect potential system points at which failure may occur, to prioritize these, and to provide alternative means of accomplishing the same goal. FMEA starts at the front end of the process and identifies potential events. FTA starts at the level of an existing process, identifies and collects data on actual failures, and works backward toward the beginning of the process with the intent of identifying opportunities for redesign.

A formula which can be used to help assess the relative effects of potential failures is

$$p = Kft \qquad\qquad (4\text{-}1)$$

where

p = Effective probability of failure
K = Severity effect of failure
    K = 0.0, negligible effect
    K = 0.1, marginal effect
    K = 0.5, critical effect
    K = 1.0, catastrophic effect
f = Frequency of occurrence, event per unit time
t = Time scale over which effect occurs

For example, assume that a process flow diagram shows that a hospital phlebotomist is scheduled to draw blood in the early hours of the morning so that daily testing can be complete and on the patients' charts before the attending physicians do their daily rounds. This isn't a total disaster if it isn't done; that is, someone can go back up and do it, but the lab instruments now have to be set up for additional runs and accessioning has a double wave of work. Thus, this misstep is arbitrarily assigned into a K = 0.5 severity class. The significance of this situation has been downplayed with the K scaling factor. This is only useful for relative rankings of the various points of system failure. In addition, the usual rules for independent events apply such that overall probability = $P(t) = p1 \times p2 \times p3 \times \ldots$ and so on. The overall system reliability = $R(t) = R1 \times R2 \times R3 \times \ldots$ and so on. All of this falls under the E part of FMEA, or the effect of system failure. It is sometimes called risk rating or relative risk rating. The M or failure mode is the symptom of failure, the indicator or measurement associated with the system breakdown at that point. This provides the guideline for data collection for the FTA.

Once the system is up and running, FTA can be used retrospectively to assess damage already done. FMEA tries to do this in a more predictive a priori sense. Either can use risk rating. The tree in FTA develops from the generation of a graphical display of errors and their cause-effect statements. See Figure 4.5 for an example using the phlebotomy incident reviewed in this section.

FMEA uses a tabular enumeration of the failure modes and their relative priorities. Using the example, Table 4.1 shows how this summary would have evolved from FMEA.

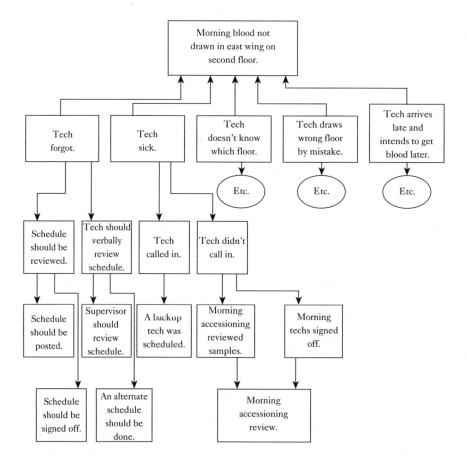

Figure 4.5: Fault tree analysis. Assuming a chronic problem occurring with the system of morning phlebotomy, the fault tree starts with known reasons for no blood drawn. In practice, these would be tabulated so that the causes for the system failure could be prioritized. The fault tree analysis then proceeds to break these down into root causes and potential additional causes so that remediation can be focused on the major causes of failure and contingency planning can accommodate these.

Table 4.1: FMEA of hospital blood collection.

Process: floor and unit morning blood collection

Component	Cause of failure	P/S*	Effect of failure	Alternatives
Phlebotomist	No show	$1/4$†	Blood delivery delayed	See FTA
Phlebotomist	Late	$1/3$	Blood delivery delayed	See FTA
Phlebotomist	Drew wrong location	$1/2$	Blood delivery delayed	See FTA

* P = Probability of occurrence; S = Seriousness of failure to system

† 1 = very low; 2 = low; 3 = medium; 4 = high; 5 = very high

Both FMEA and FTA eventually generate statements for remediation and improvement. These are listed on the process decision program chart. The quality improvement committee will want to review these statements for incorporation into the process flowchart for completeness. The PDPC can look like the FTA diagram or the FMEA table, but the overall purpose is to identify those steps of the process which may periodically fail and to develop contingency plans to minimize the failure based on the relative impact that such a failure has on the process.

Matrix Diagram

The matrix diagram is one of the most helpful planning tools because of its applicability to simple as well as complex situations. There are several types of matrix diagrams (T-shaped, L-shaped, integrated), and they are all used to explore the relationship between two operations. Juran shows the L-shaped diagram used in quality function deployment as relating customer needs to plant output, and then relating plant output to system design for that output and control of the system.[1] Figure 4.6 shows the matrix diagram integrating customer needs to lab output, and Figure 4.7 shows the matrix diagram applied to the lab reporting operation.

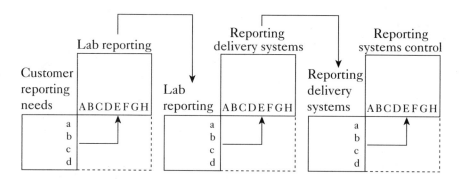

Figure 4.6: The matrix diagram—integrating customer needs to lab output. This matrix diagram is used to integrate the customer's needs to the laboratory's control system for generating and delivering reports.

The diagram is made by putting market issues (customer needs) on the left margin and the laboratory delivery on the top. These are arranged in columns and lines and a mark is placed at the intersection if there is a correlation between the customer needs and the lab effort to meet these needs. The mark may be of several types. Any mark at all would identify correlation. For instance, one hospital may set the lab delivery system at "issue legible reports." The customer need is "reports to chart by 7:00 A.M." At the intersection of this need/delivery, a mark for correlation would be put, but it wouldn't indicate complete satisfaction of the customer's needs. It would be an opportunity for improvement.

In much of the Japanese literature, the symbols for the relative impact of the correlation are given by the target, circle, and triangle which are the Japanese horse racing symbols for win, place, and show. This results in a coarse ranking of how well the correlations meet. More detailed information can be obtained by using numerical rankings of the three discriminator classes (see Figure 4.8).

Matrix Data Analysis

This technique is the planning equivalent of design of experiments and multivariate analysis. It requires data collection and a computer-assisted summary analysis. The process uses a technique called principal component analysis and results in some rather complicated visual displays of correlations. Again if the resources are available then use this analysis. If not, better return can be obtained with more prudent efforts elsewhere. The genius of Deming and Juran was to bring some very difficult concepts to line-level use. The fact that some of them are now evolving away from the line is a reflection of the sophistication of the

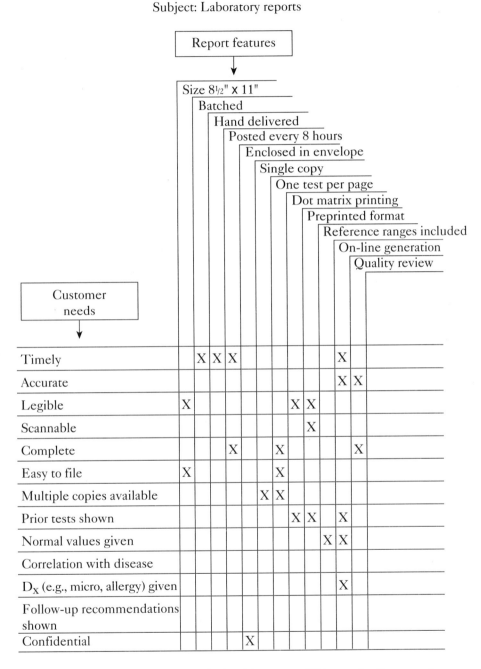

Figure 4.7: Matrix diagram applied to lab reports. This matrix diagram relates customer needs in the reporting area to the laboratory's capabilities in reporting. The X's represent correlation. Scanning from left to right, the more X's the better. Where there are no X's (correlation with disease, follow-up), there is no current lab offering which meets the customer's need.

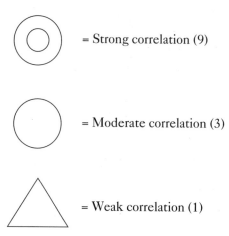

Figure 4.8: Correlation symbols. These symbols are used in various matrix diagrams to indicate the degree of correlation between one axis and the other. The symbols are derived from the Japanese horse racing marks for win, place, and show.

companies which are using the concepts and evidence of the companies' commitment to this effort.

Systematic Diagram

This is also called the dendrogram or tree diagram. It is a technique used to systematically study a process in increasing detail until root causes are revealed for each of the process characteristics. Alternately, the technique can be used to break down a process improvement method into finer steps until all sequential stages are identified for the transformation.

Figure 4.9 shows a systematic diagram which illustrates the deployment of policy management. The systematic diagram, if detailed, would represent the steps in accomplishing this deployment in finer and finer detail as the processes are passed on down from the planning levels to the operational levels.

Arrow Diagram

The arrow diagram is used to define and analyze a specific plan when all the steps and their relative sequences are known. The arrow diagram comes from operations research (OR) and shares some commonality with the PERT and critical path method (CPM). Whereas many OR people correctly point out that PERT/CPM offer advantages over the Gantt chart in terms of project description, the Gantt chart is simple and easily understood.

The arrow diagram has some advantages: it can focus on the sequencing of the steps in the plan; it can show concurrent processes; and it can

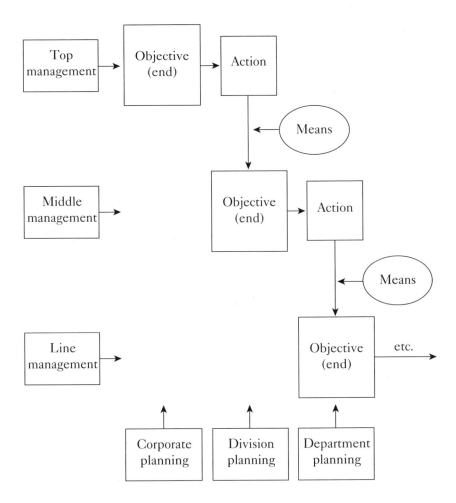

Figure 4.9: Responsibilities in policy management—a systematic diagram. This systematic diagram outlines the roles of different management levels and different business levels in the deployment of policy management. Effective policy management always provides the means to an end, or the plan by means of which an objective is achieved. This is in contrast to traditional management by objective which sets goals, but frequently leaves the attainment of these goals up to the ingenuity of the individual given the responsibility of attaining them.

streamline processes by eliminating redundant steps. The arrow diagram, however, is not for the neophyte. Software exists to help in the effort.

Brief Summary of the Seven New Tools

Both the affinity diagram and the relationship diagram are used to identify, organize, and conceptualize complex problems with multiple associations. The matrix diagram, matrix data analysis, and the systematic diagram are used to reduce these complex interrelationships to more manageable forms and to provide some structure relating these concepts to material action and control processes and plans. The PDPC is used to analyze and structure contingency mechanisms for proposed plans. Arrow diagrams are used to provide a path forward; they are the detailed means by which the plans may be implemented.

ROOT CAUSE ANALYSIS

Root cause analysis is a technique used to determine the main causes which contribute to a process output. Root cause analysis assumes a cause-and-effect relationship between process outcome and the root cause. One technique also allows for identification of root effects; that is, the primary effects of the root cause. This technique uses the affinity diagram and the relationship diagram.

The affinity diagram is completed by brainstorming the subject matter. In Figure 4.10 the subject was "What is causing difficulty in introducing TQM to your facility?" The brainstorming activity resulted in six areas of related subject matter, and these were used as input for the relationship diagram. In completing the relationship diagram, arrows are drawn from cause to effect. To start the diagram, an arrow is drawn from each of the subjects to the initial question which is centered within the diagram. This identifies what was originally asked, so that each subject should indeed be a separate cause of the central issue. Each of the affinity diagram groups should cause problems in introducing TQM.

Next, starting with any of the groups, an arrow is drawn to each of the other subjects which the chosen group affects. For instance, employee resistance would affect the introduction of TQM. It would also affect general company disinterest, since employees are a large part of the company. It wouldn't affect no employee input, no training, high cost of TQM, or senior management apathy. When this operation is finished, the component is scored by counting the number of arrows in and the number of arrows out. This summary for the entire diagram is shown in Table 4.2.

The component with the highest number of arrows going out is the root cause—it affects more of the related components. The component with the most number of arrows going in is the root effect—it is affected by more of the other components.

This analysis helps to determine where company efforts should go to arrive at a solution to the problem. For instance, when the problem is

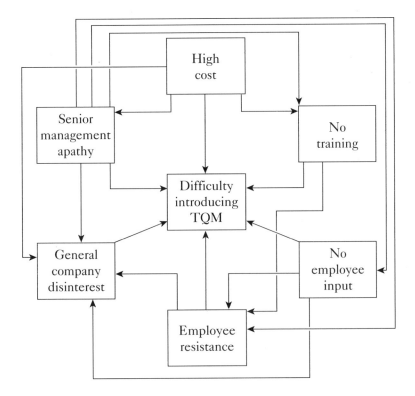

Figure 4.10: Relationship diagram, root cause analysis. This is a relationship diagram from an affinity diagram that resulted in six related groups. The question posed to the task group was "What is causing difficulty in introducing TQM to your facility?" The relationship diagram used the output of the affinity diagram and explored the cause-and-effect relationship between the affinity diagram headings. In this way the root cause was identified as senior management apathy, and the root effect was identified as general company disinterest.

identified and the affinity diagram is completed, it would have been easy to say that the real problem with the company is a general disinterest. Thus, to turn this attitude around, the company should invest a lot of money in marketing TQM internally, perhaps with slogans, games, incentives, and so on. The relationship diagram, however, identified general company disinterest as a root effect, and consequently, no amount of effort will turn around the company until senior management, who is the real spectre at the feast, turns around its own attitude and begins to overtly demonstrate support for the TQM effort. This, in turn, will save the company a great deal of wasted time and effort barking up the wrong tree.

Table 4.2: Summary of relationship diagram.

	Arrows		
Component	*Out*	*In*	
Senior management apathy	5	1	(Root cause)
High cost	4	0	
No employee input	3	1	
No training	2	2	
Employee resistance	2	3	
General company disinterest	1	4	(Root effect)

Note here that two of the new seven planning tools were used, and this example illustrates their utility in helping to solve problems of considerable scope. The QC tools could have been used, again starting with brainstorming to generate the bones of an Ishikawa diagram. Since this is a cause-and-effect diagram, the causes of difficulty in implementing TQM are explored. In Figure 4.11, a fishbone diagram is shown in which the main bones are derived from brainstorming. If the original 6-M bones were used, machine, measurement, and materials, would have been immediately discarded, and men (people, personnel), milieu (environmental factors), and methods would have been explored. Note that with the exception of cost, all of the other factors are people related.

This exercise helps to show the difference between using the tools for problem solving, of which root cause analysis is a part, and process analysis and design, which would use a fishbone up front as a sort of checklist to make certain that all aspects of a process had been considered. If the question had been, "How will we introduce TQM to our facility?" then all of the bones in the fishbone would be addressed routinely. For instance, since in-house training may not have been a large part of the previous management style, there may not be any on-site facility to do training. Perhaps the cafeteria must be set up auditorium-style each time a training session is scheduled. Facilities maintenance might find this a real inconvenience and plans to assess the lab a hefty interdepartmental charge for it. This would appear under the milieu (environmental) bone and would be addressed as part of the process design. The way the problem is stated, though, the participants identified aspects of the problem which targeted management as being the root cause.

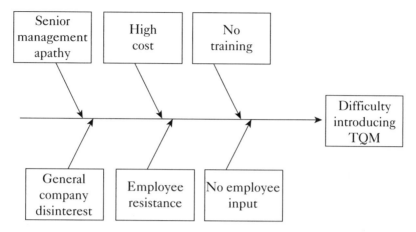

Figure 4.11: Ishikawa diagram, root cause analysis. This fishbone diagram was derived from brainstorming which identified the six categories shown. If the brainstorming activity included the generation of an affinity diagram, most of the little bones would also have been identified.

Note that all six components which came from the affinity diagram, which generated the relationship diagram, can be thought of as causes of the effect, and this is why they can be plugged back into the fishbone. Note also that if senior management apathy could be removed as a root cause, then cost would replace it as the key regressive factor. In this sense the relationship diagram may help to prioritize the causes which result in the process output. With regard to cost, establishing this as a primary cause of lack of response to TQM initiatives would require some special insights. First, the category probably should have been labeled perceived costs because the underlying message of Deming and Juran is that lack of quality is what costs, and even Crosby captured this so well in *Quality Is Free*. Second, the issue of costs is always of paramount importance even in the issue of root cause determination. For instance, just as Pareto techniques reveal where the best investment of time would be for process improvement, a financial Pareto would reveal the maximum return for the minimum investment. So the prioritization takes place in two steps, the first identifying the root cause and the components of the root cause, and the second integrating these with financial resources to identify which areas will yield the most return on the dollar invested.

This section provides an example of using the tools in a fashion fitting to the problem, opportunity, or situation. The next chapter looks at the concepts of process analysis, process improvement, and tool use in more detail.

NOTE

1. J. M. Juran, *Juran on Leadership for Quality: An Executive Handbook* (New York: Free Press, 1989), 119.

SUGGESTED READING

Gitlow, Howard S., and Process Management International. *Planning for Quality, Productivity, and Competitive Position*. Homewood, Ill.: Richard D. Irwin, 1990.

Mizuno, Shigeru. *Management for Quality Improvement: The Seven New QC Tools*. Cambridge, Mass.: Productivity Press, 1988.

5

Using TQM Tools to Effect Process Improvement

Having mastered the basics of the seven quality tools and the new seven planning tools, the next step is using these in an organized way. The TQM way is known as the QC story. This is a seven-step method which identifies process improvements consistent with management policy, analyzes them, and then implements them. In addition, the QC story documents the process improvement activities. In this way, the quality improvement process proceeds in an organized, reproducible direction, and the documentation is used to teach those who follow what went on in the analytical process. Organizing and archiving this process improvement data is not a trivial task, and arranging it so that it is easily retrieved and used is an issue which must be addressed early.

This improvement process is called kaizen, and perhaps the best review of it is in Masaaki Imai's book, *Kaizen*. Imai shows how pervasive the entire concept of kaizen is to the Japanese culture. The process of Kaizen begins with individuals and includes their personal life, social life, and business and professional life. This basic philosophy then extends into the culture to include various group activities in which the concept of kaizen plays

131

a basic role. To find it in the industrial setting, then, is a natural extension of this personal perspective into the Japanese business world.

The process itself is most clearly seen in Figure 5.1 which outlines the process. A more detailed procedure adapted from a Minneapolis-based group called Process Management International (PMI) is shown as Figure 5.2. This breaks down the seven major steps into sub-processes with clarifying remarks on each step. The steps are based on the Deming wheel, the PDCA cycle. The planning part of the cycle includes the first three steps, followed by the limited deployment in step 4, the check cycle in step 5, and succeeded by complete deployment, standardization, and chronicling.

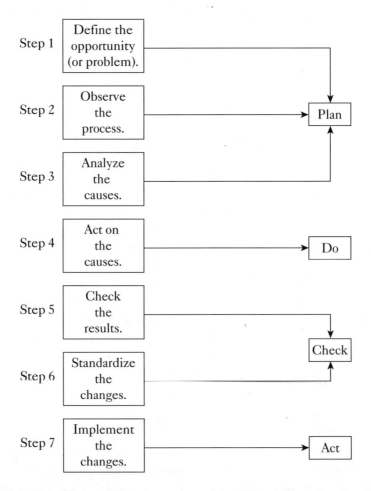

Figure 5.1: The QC story. The seven steps of the QC story are related to the Deming wheel. The QC story is a way to formally effect process change and record the way it was done.

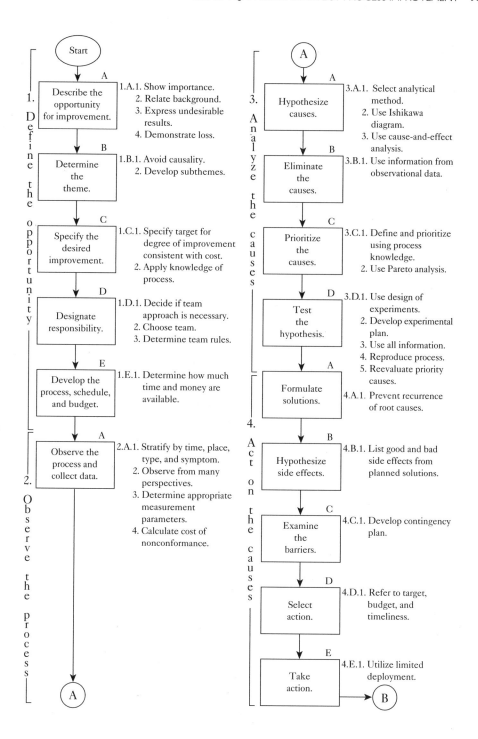

Figure 5.2: Flowchart for process improvement. The QC story.

continued

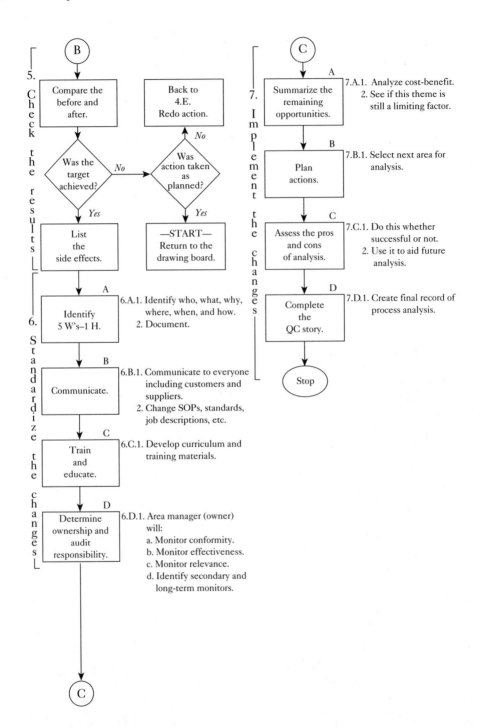

Figure 5.2: *continued*

DEFINE THE PROBLEM

The distance between what a process is delivering and what the process should be delivering is known as a performance gap, or simply the gap. In the West this is viewed in a positive sense, as an opportunity for improvement; the Japanese view it as a problem. The problem is "Why aren't we doing better?" "How can we make the process better?" "Where can we improve?" "How can we do better?" "What are we doing wrong?" "How soon can we improve this?"

The first step in analyzing for process improvement is to identify the opportunities for improvement. This begins with a flowchart of the system. The Japanese have a saying—Quality begins and ends with training. The process improvement method begins and ends with a flowchart. The flowchart gives a pictorial view of the process and helps to focus efforts on the process and to clearly define it. Dissection begins here with an analysis of the process steps. Be careful to note any unnecessary steps.

At this point the process history and background should be evaluated. In essence, this is the why of the process. To further understand the relationship of the process to the overall department effort, the supply and delivery sides of the process should be reviewed. What does the process deliver, or to whom or what department is the service provided? On the front end, what is the impetus for the process start? What causes the process to activate?

Carefully define the gap. What is the process currently delivering? What should the process deliver? The difference is the performance shortfall. In addition, costs become a consideration—the cost of noncompliance and the cost of change. The latter becomes clear in this planning process as the project outlines are explicitly defined.

Choose a new process improvement team or redirect a current analytical group. As is discussed in the section on plan implementation, the company should have in place a structure for evaluating and enabling process improvement teams including a tracking and review process. The management structure acknowledges and records the subject of review as well as conveys prior approval and support. Address this step in keeping with company policy.

Create a Gantt chart or alternative method for tracking and projecting the process improvement steps and associated costs. This is another visual organizer of notable value. At this point the initial planning efforts are largely done and it is time to make certain that all team members have actually seen the process in action.

OBSERVE THE PROCESS

The process improvement group will have on it individuals intimately associated with the process as it currently runs. Additional members may come from the supply or delivery side of the process, and still others may come from the executive, managerial, or staffing positions. The degree of familiarity with the process for team members will vary greatly. Despite the intimacy that some members have for the process, the team members should all observe the process as it is ongoing. This should take place from the several perspectives in which the team members have expertise. It may be viewed from a cost standpoint, an efficiency or industrial engineering view, the harmony of the alignment between supplier or user and the system operation, and environmental and safety positions.

This is a good place to use a well-designed check sheet which can standardize points which all members should comment on and review from their individual perspectives. The process should also be observed during different times (shifts, for instance) and on occasions when it is likely to be optimum, and others when it is not. For instance, this would be holidays, weekends, and periods of short staff such as breaks, lunch hour, and so on. Remember the idea is not that the current process is a disaster, but that the goal is improvement. Improvement may simply be to shore up an already good process in its moments of weakness.

After all the observations, the views are shared and discussion of the measurement parameters begins. The group must decide which characteristics of the process warrant quantification, or if they are even amenable to measurement processes, or if alternative ways such as according subjective impressions a quantitative aspect, need to be employed. This is a critical component and may be subject to modification as the analysis continues. The point is that the process delivers something of importance, or that it shouldn't continue and the process delivery requires a reduction to measurable output. Alternatively the process may be comprised of subsystems which directly relate to the overall system performance, and these may be used to quantify the process output. A direct correlation must at least be inferred between the measurement and the process delivery, however, or the measurable output won't reflect change whether good or bad, in the process. This is one of the fail-safe ingredients of TQM and to overlook it is to ask for trouble by way of introducing process change with no sense of whether or not the change is beneficial.

ANALYZE THE CAUSES

Here is where the prior work with the seven quality tools and the management tools is brought in. The analytical process consists of brainstorming for contributing causes to the process variability, and this can be done conventionally or by using the affinity diagram.

The causes are then put on the Ishikawa diagram under the 6-M headings. Parenthetically, the bones can be anything, but the 6-M headings are useful in generating ideas and starting the group output. The point is, don't confine the group to these as the sole issues. They are used simply because they are basic and common to most processes.

Causes are then prioritized using Pareto analysis. Prior to this, some causes may be eliminated based on the earlier observation step in which some causes may be viewed by the group as irrelevant.

Pareto analysis is best done when causes are prioritized using actual relevant data. Remember Pareto's principle is the 80/20 rule that 80 percent of the process variation is a result of 20 percent of the causes. Data collection can help confirm this or at least identify major contributors, providing that brainstorming and cause-and-effect diagrams have truly included the root causes and not just symptomatology.

To determine this, design of experiments can be employed in which the selected causes can be varied in a planned fashion. Properly done, causality may be inferred from the outcome analysis. At the end of this, it is time to summarize the main causes and develop a plan of action.

ACT ON THE CAUSES

This may sound fairly straightforward. Having progressed this far, the causes of process variability should be identified, and fixing the process is simply eliminating the variation. Removing the causes may not be quite as simple as this. Sometimes there are real barriers to doing this. For instance, the funds, equipment, or trained personnel may not be available. In addition, the root cause removal may have undesirable side effects which complicate a related process. These must be fit into the overall picture and weighed in the balance with remediation.

Having done this, various solutions to the problem have differing degrees of appeal. These can be analyzed using force-field analysis, or if the resources are available, matrix data analysis. Having selected the course of action, it is time to deploy it on a limited scale.

CHECK THE RESULTS

The check cycle is a key feature of Deming management. It has its source rooted in the scientific method and reflects the origins of the founders of Japanese TQC. It is also the fundamental feature that makes TQM different from other management ideologies which have structured methods for developing policies and setting them in place. The check cycle automatically sets a prior requirement for the determination of system variables which relate to the process performance. It also includes a measurement of the system delivery. Without these, the check cycle has nothing to check. In most other systems this is the primary weakness inasmuch as policies are deployed with no subsequent monitoring of their effect on the system.

The check cycle requires a measurement of the effect of the implemented change on the system performance. There may be more than one reason why the change hasn't showed positive effect. For instance, the wrong root causes may have been chosen for removal or alteration. The wrong measurement variable may have been chosen to reflect the system delivery. Whatever the case, if the subsequent measurements in the check cycle indicate that improvement, as viewed by the recipient of the process delivery, hasn't occurred to the extent anticipated, then the flowchart indicates a return to the planning cycle for a rethink of the strategy. If, on the other hand, progress has taken place, then it is time to move into the act cycle of the Deming wheel. Figure 5.3 on method design reflects the steps to this point.

STANDARDIZE THE CHANGES

The questions, why, when, where, who, what, and how, must be addressed in the act cycle and another Gantt chart, this time for full-scale implementation, should be prepared. The SOPs are done in keeping with the regulatory environment and distributed for review and sign-off.

At this point another key feature of TQM is the identification of the process owner, generally the manager of the area in which the process

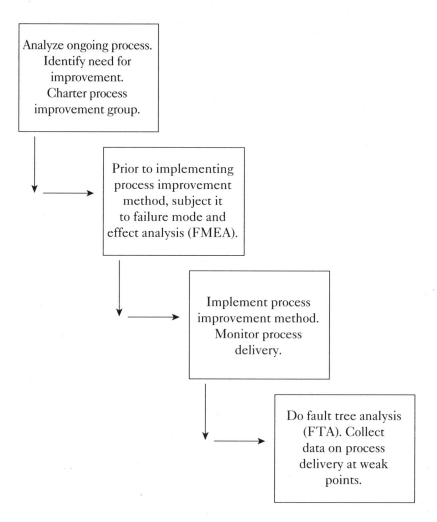

Figure 5.3: Method design and critique. In developing a process improvement method, generation and deployment of the process are only part of the overall scheme. The process must be subjected to FMEA prior to deployment, with the intent of assessing the method with regard to potential weaknesses. This is done most effectively by another group separate from the original process design group. Following deployment, the process delivery is monitored, and the process shortcomings are assessed by means of FTA.

occurs. Juran cautions that it is the job of the process owner to make certain that the process delivery stays at the new level of performance. It is done by the owner's constant monitoring of the performance. Nothing short of constant vigilance for the well-being of the new process will do. It must be nurtured and helped along. This is an internal check cycle within the act cycle. Again, it is inherent in TQM. The major reason for TQM failure is inadequate review. In addition to the monitoring by the process owner, secondary review should be instituted with its own schedule. This will include external review such as from a quality assurance department and senior management.

Communication to all departments and individuals who play a role in the new and improved process takes place at this point. "Quality begins and ends with training," says Imai, and this is the time to believe it and take action based on this teaching.

IMPLEMENT CHANGES

A date and time for the process change is set, and the change begun by all departments and people party to it. This is almost the easy part, at least for the planning group, because the responsibility for the change and monitoring has been relayed to the line people who will make it happen. It remains for the process improvement group to review the pros and cons of the improvement operation and to document the process as it actually happened. This is important for the benefit of those who will follow; those working on similar processes and analyzing them in a similar way. It is a learning component of TQM.

As a final formality, the process improvement group will make recommendations for future functions which subsequent planning groups will want to address as priorities indicate the need. A use of the QC story in process malfunction is shown in Figure 5.4.

SUMMARY REMARKS

Gitlow refers to the process improvement method as the "atom" of TQM. By this he means that it is the irreducible minimum, or the building block, from which the rest of the structure can be formed. This process is best represented by the flowchart or by a flowchart which represents the process improvement as illustrated in the QC story. The entire thrust of TQM is the continual improvement of existing processes by a rational method using the QC and management tools. In thinking about this, picture the process as a forward-moving force and the process improvement method as an upward-moving force which brings the existing process more into line with the anticipated delivery of the new and improved system. This is illustrated in Figure 5.5.

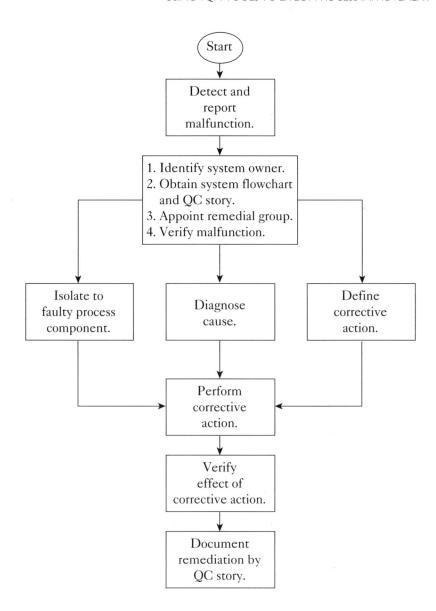

Figure 5.4: Correcting a process malfunction. The use of the QC story in remedying a process malfunction is portrayed.

QUALITY FUNCTION DEPLOYMENT

The Voice of the Customer

Quality function deployment (QFD) is uniquely Japanese. Developed in the Mitsubishi shipyards, it is the key to integrating the voice of the customer into company quality goals. In Japan, if the customer wants a bicycle, the buyer sits on a form which takes individual measurements for

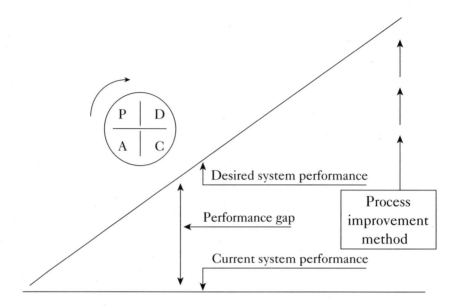

Figure 5.5: Method and process improvement. The performace gap is the observable difference between the current system performance and the desired system performance. The performance gap is closed using the process improvement method described by the flowchart generated in the QC story.

leg length, arm position and extension, and a number of other personal preferences. These are sent to the factory electronically where they are reduced to a computer input driving an assembly line which produces the custom-designed bike in two days. The Japanese add a nice touch by holding delivery of the bike for two weeks to let the anticipation grow. This shows the extent which the Japanese now go to personalize the delivery of service and product. This individualizing of services and product has become a recent addition to the Japanese process delivery philosophy.

Understanding the Customer's Requirements

QFD begins with a market-in attitude and business culture as opposed to the traditional product-out orientation. Businesses have long been run under the assumption that the businesses would create new products or services, introduce the public to them, and the novelty of the offering would assure the success of the venture. This reasoning is appropriate for a fledgling service, one which the public hasn't seen and which fills a previously empty niche. It is not appropriate for a mature service offering such as the clinical laboratory. In mature service segments, the buyer discriminates based on the quality of service delivered, if the price is the same as others. In the clinical lab, however, service is the same and price is the discriminator. In addition, the price charged for the service is frequently not borne by the buyer, but underwritten by taxpayers through Medicare and Medicaid or by insurance companies. As indicated earlier, even though pricing is fairly uniform throughout the industry, a condition brought about by considerable direct competition, TQM can make a lab much more profitable than its competitors by decreasing fixed and variable costs achieved by increasing efficiency in process delivery. QFD, on the other hand, increases market share through identifying and satisfying customer wants.

Noriaki Kano refers to "specified quality" as the delivery of products or services which the customer has identified as being key to his or her basic contentment. This Kano calls a "satisfier." Committing to this level of service is, in essence, the marketing equivalent of Maslow's criteria. Satisfiers are necessary to maintain market share. They fulfill the customer's needs. This is good, because prior to QFD, businesses were delivering what they thought the customer wanted. So a satisfier is good, but the quality effort must deliver better than this to increase market share.

In the clinical lab, the customer has seldom been asked what he or she wants in the line of service. So to identify and deliver this routinely is a very big step. The client has both implied and implicit needs. Implicit needs are those which the customer truly has to have to deliver satisfaction. The implied needs are those which address additional perceived requirements which the client believes would make doing business with the lab easy. In this latter category, trained salespeople are taught to identify which of these implied needs are critical to closing the sale. In effect they are doing a mental Pareto analysis and trying to identify the handful of requirements which the client has identified as decisive and offering to deliver these in return for the client's business. Formally this is known as needs analysis.

Using QFD, businesses try to determine which of all the client-identified needs are important to maintain the existing business, to prioritize these, and to develop systems to enhance the delivery of these important service components. In effect, businesses use the sales closing as an initial data source on which to draw information on customer requirements. There are, of course, many ongoing means by which businesses continue to tap clientele needs. Deming believes that this is critical to maintaining the vitality of the TQM establishment. Deming views any consumer base as a market which is constantly changing. He also believes that businesses must be constantly sensitive to the changing needs of the market and to have internal systems which are able to quickly respond to the changing needs of the marketplace.

There is, however, a problem with simply delivering at this basic service level. A certain amount of time the reverse of a satisfier, the dissatisfier, is generated. This considerably outweighs the service counterparts. Though a dissatisfier is delivered much less frequently, its impact is much greater. The customer comes to take the service for granted. Day in and day out the customer sees the same routine quality effort. It is known that satisfied customers may tell two to three others of their contentment. Dissatisfied customers will always tell many times this number.

When a dissatisfier is inadvertently produced, the client is alienated and calls to squawk about it. This is good. Surveys say that the customer who calls and complains is most likely to stay with the business which has aggravated him or her, particularly if the customer has a legitimate complaint which is addressed and rectified by the establishment. The client which is most likely to be lost is the one who suffers in silence and finally moves on in hopes of finding something better elsewhere. The business must access this customer and find out his or her views through QFD.

Kano recommends delivering a degree of service over and above that which is identified as a requirement by the customer. These he piquantly calls "delighters" or "exciters." These categories of service commitment come from within the company, from the ingenuity and creativity of the marketing group. Consequently, the company must foster and encourage avenues for implementing the creative process. This can lead to quantum improvement in the delivery of the service component.

Imai says that the Japanese originally understood the PDCA cycle, as taught by Deming, to be directed at integrating research and engineering design with production and sales using quality as a central focus. Following Juran's definition of quality as "fitness for use," it fell to the Japanese to find a method for linking the customer's voice to the design of the product or service through QFD.

The Language of Sales

The purpose of language is communication. According to linguists, there is no standard or benchmark English. Reference to the King's English means that, when in the court, it is best to use that particular dialect and usage, but it won't do in the Bronx or a similar urban locale. In the Bronx, if you want to communicate well and to garner local acceptance, it is best to employ Bronx English usage. You can be in or you can be out, and the language you use may control this.

In the preliterate stage of the evolution of language, grunts, hand signs, and facial and body expressions would have sufficed to convey the limited meanings and messages of a simpler time. To an extent human beings still carry this in the form of body language. Body language can convey strong emotional meaning.

Early on, a grunt and a hand sign may have meant, "Grog, you circle that mammoth to the right and stab it with your spear, hoping to kill it. I will organize the party to cut up and distribute the meat."

At some point Grog may have grunted back, "You stab the (ancient expletive deleted) Mammoth." This would have led to the evolution of a more complex form of dialogue in order to convey the idea that "If you stab the mammoth, Grog, then you will gain much stature in the community and be known as a brave and fearless man." Persuasion could initially be done by force, but later, verbal skills would be needed to convince. Enter the sales representative.

Figure 5.6 shows the correspondence between sales and QFD. The sales function is to generate new customers. The QFD function is primarily to keep the current customers. A secondary function of QFD is to generate new customers through referrals effected by the enhanced company image as viewed by happy consumers.

The seven-step process of selling begins with the identification of the individual responsible for the purchase. This is critical because people don't like admitting that they don't have responsibility. So a salesperson can waste considerable time delivering a presentation to the wrong person, only to learn on closing that the individual doesn't have the authority to make the decision.

After making certain that the presentation is delivered on target, the salesperson must deduce what the potential buyer thinks is important—the things that will interest the buyer in doing business with the salesperson's company. These take on various degrees of importance, and the salesperson must do a needs analysis, a mental prioritization of the customer's needs, to determine which and how many of them are crucial to turning the sale. If the salesperson can deliver these, then closing is simply a matter of offering these needs convincingly. The buyer should sign up unless he or she doesn't have the authority to do so.

In the seven-step, QFD parallel to this process, the company must identify representative customer voices to learn from them what is important for them to continue doing business with the company. As in the sales process, this is followed by understanding customer concerns and prioritizing them with regard to key deliverable service improvements designed to keep the customer with the company and away from the competition.

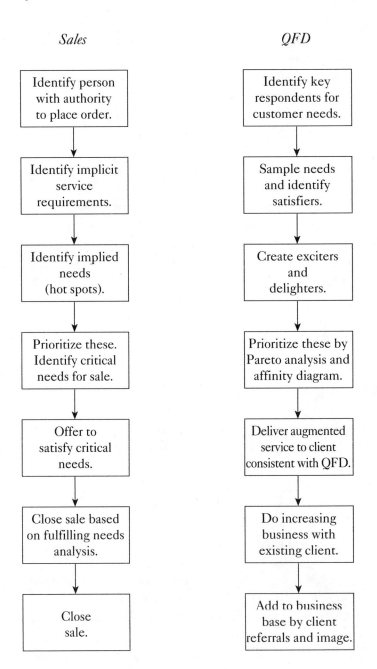

Figure 5.6: Sales and QFD.

One way to hear the customer's voice is through the focus session. The focus session is frequently used by diagnostic manufacturers to learn what users may want in the way of new equipment or diagnostic kits. The idea is to integrate customer views with product design. The focus session shares certain items in common with the sales presentation.

The focus session and the sales presentation are different in the following respects. In the focus session all individuals related to the process attend but do not focus on the short-term aspects of the sales review. The people are asked to adopt a more global view rather than a self-centered one. The focus session setting is nonthreatening and casual, and all participants contribute. In the brainstorming session, sometimes the quietest members have the best ideas since they tend to be analytical. In the sales presentation similar people attend but they are used to reinforce the presenter and to answer questions of the potential client in their area of expertise. The sales presentation, however, will eventually result in the offer of a customized service without necessarily accommodating some of the more far-reaching aspects of the service component which may not be able to be reliably delivered. The salesperson has only one goal: to close the sale and collect the commission. This attitude doesn't always integrate well with the quality effort. For this reason, salespeople are initially the most reluctant to join in the TQM effort since they tend to view the early training and reorientation as one more obstacle between themselves and the sale. This training takes time away from them which they feel could better be used on the phone or on sales calls.

After the TQM effort has been successfully deployed, the salespeople will be the most supportive and appreciative of it. They will find that they now are able to make sales easier, to guarantee the client a service level with a greater level of confidence, and to present the potential client with concrete credentials of performance, as well as references of other happy customers. Of all the people who transform during the deployment of TQM, the salespeople are the most fun to watch.

In the focus session there is generally only a brief presentation followed by very general leading questions. At this juncture the facilitator has no clear guidance of where the ideas are going to take the group. The meeting is lead by a facilitator who must be very sharp, one who must know all aspects of the process under review in order to evaluate whether answers are complete or well directed. For instance, if the group includes a technical component, the facilitator must be able to evaluate technical input for suitability.

Diagnostic manufacturers use focus sessions to integrate customer needs to product design. Currently, this is generally done after the product is designed, and it is used to assess suitability retrospectively. The key to estimating the users' attitudes is to be very cautious about leading them down the path which the manufacturer's natural bias would like them to proceed. Sometimes, however, the group won't make the intellectual jump to the level of the new product idea, in which case the manufacturer will want to share more details with the group in order to get feedback on issues which may never have been raised. This is a reminder of Deming's cautionary statement; that although the client will respond clearly to needs regarding process improvement, he or she will rarely, if ever, invent the components needed for process breakthrough.

COMPARING DEMING'S SALES
AND DESIGN INTEGRATION WITH QFD

Deming suggested integrating the customer's views into design in a way that would consolidate all company functions into focusing on a market-in orientation. He envisioned this being done in a production setting by linking the following business functions: customer requirements, design requirements, part characteristics, production requirements, and manufacturing operations. As shown in Table 5.1, this can be easily translated into the service setting by understanding to what the individual components refer. The example in Table 5.1 uses the reporting function to show how the lab links customer reporting requirements into the operational flow stream.

Following Juran, the customer needs can be linked to the lab operation by means of the matrix diagram. Juran views this as a three-part process whereby the linkage is achieved between the process customer needs, the lab systems to supply those needs, and the control functions on the lab systems (see Figure 4.6). In this fashion, through three coupled matrix diagrams, the customer needs are linked to control functions which minimize the system variation which responds to these needs. In addition, this process prioritizes the system components which most closely relate to the delivery of the specified needs. This streamlines the delivery system and results in a clean response. The resultant system is one free of extraneous components only loosely related to the customer requirements.

This prioritization function can be clarified using a very simple matrix diagram. The diagram has few components to show how the establishment of these priorities is done. This technique is used in many places in TQM

Table 5.1: Lab reporting, QFD integration.

Customer requirement	Return reports
Design requirements	How often
	How to do it
	• Courier
	• Mail
	• Fax
	• Electronic
	• Database
	Billing cross-check
Part characteristics	Envelope (content, bill)
	Report
	• Format
	• What information
	• Size, appearance
	• Patient concerns
	• Customization
Production requirements	Match to design
Manufacturing operations	Where, when, who, what

to establish, clarify, and rank relationships. It will be used again in chapter 7, where the corporate mission and long-term goals are linked with departmental systems and goals established by this same process.

The House of Quality

The house of quality is a name given to the matrix diagram developed in 1972 at the Mitsubishi shipyards in Kobe, Japan. The matrix diagram originally had a peak on the top which was the result of an additional correlation. This gave the diagram a houselike look, and so the Japanese called it the house of quality. What the diagram does is to semiquantitatively link customer needs with business output capabilities and to prioritize opportunities for improvement in correlation between what the customer wants and what the business delivers. It is unlikely in the lab operation that the full-blown QFD diagram will be used to any great extent, but the concept behind what it is doing needs to be understood conceptually.

A schematic of the QFD house of quality is given in Figure 5.7. The customer needs are listed on the left. These are converted into company quality characteristics, sometimes referred to as substitute quality characteristics. These appear in the upper part of the matrix. This transla-tion occurs because the customer will frequently express wants in a fash-ion which doesn't directly relate to the business output. A characteristic such as "wants a legible report" can be reflected in a number of different ways from the perspective of the lab. It is also necessary to find out what legible really means to the account. The paper may be too thin and so ear-lier reports from the patient record show through from below. Perhaps the print quality generated from a dot-matrix printer isn't clear enough. Perhaps it is clear until the ribbon wears down to where it isn't clear any longer. Maybe the typeface chosen is too small or too unusual for quick reading.

All of these things translate into the business substitute characteristics as type of paper, type of font, and type of printer, and lead to a business plan which incorporates these concerns in a rational fashion. It may also lead

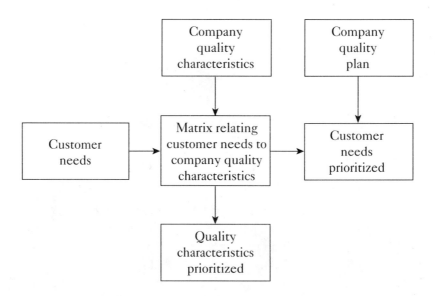

Figure 5.7: QFD matrix. Quality function deployment (QFD) relates the voice of the customer to the voice of the business. Through the QFD matrix the customer needs are prioritized in keeping with the business' ability to respond to these needs. This results in prioritizing company quality characteristics. This analysis allows management to focus the finite company resources in the areas identified by the customer as most needing response. It also allows the business to begin plan-ning for response to secondary areas in which internal resources are suboptimal.

to a search for a better paper at a good price, and a switch from a dot-matrix to a laser printer. One way in which these substitute characteristics lead to a plan is by showing the correlation in the body of the matrix using the correlation symbols shown in Figure 4.8. These are one set of correlation symbols currently in common use. The seminal article on QFD in this country by Hauser and Clausing mentions several others.[2] The idea is to see whether the customer need is addressed well or poorly by the current business capability. If the correlation between the need and the delivery is good, then the correlation is high, and there may be less of a need to respond. If the correlation is weak and the priority is identified as being high, then a response is in order.

In this example, the individual reading the report is the customer. It could have equally well been an internal customer, the next person down in an integrated system of process delivery. QFD works in either case. To learn more about the details of QFD the interested reader is referred to the book by Dr. Vincent Omachonu.[3] Not only is the example given a health care related one, the matrix diagram is modernized and each step in the QFD process is carefully described. For the purposes here, it is important to understand the concept of integrating the customer voice into the business delivery and capability, and being able to prioritize a plan for this. This technique was referenced earlier (Figure 4.7), and it will be used again later.

SPINAL FLUID CYCLE TIME: ANALYSIS OF A HOSPITAL PROCESS

Problem statement: The cycle time for analytical testing of spinal fluid specimens occasionally exceeds the standards set by the medical director.

Discussion

The hospital clinical laboratory tests many different kinds of specimens which are sent in from the nursing stations. These include blood, serum, plasma, urine, stool, and culture materials. The time it takes to process these specimens was traditionally called the TAT, and recently the cycle time. The lab must be particularly meticulous in handling the spinal fluid specimen because it is one of the most difficult to get and one of the most inconvenient to redraw. Whereas many of the other test specimens are quite stable and contain analytes which are amenable to storage and batch testing, the spinal fluid specimen is more fragile. Spinal fluid may contain both red and white blood cells, which in plasma would be fairly stable. In spinal fluid, however, the tonicity is not compatible with cell survival so the cells must be counted quickly. This is done in the hematology department. There are also no preservatives in a spinal fluid draw so measured glucose concentrations will quickly decline. Glucose and other analytes are measured in the chemistry department. Additionally, the microbiology department needs an unentered specimen of its own to check for pathogenic organisms. Normal spinal fluid is sterile. The microbial testing is not included as part of this study, but the hematology and chemistry cycle times form a part of the appraisal. Although the ultimate user of these services is the attending physician, the performance standard has been set by the medical director, and this is: The longest TAT of hematology or chemistry is ≤90 minutes.

The reason for this specification is that hematology and chemistry do their work nearly concurrently and report results to the nursing floor by computor link. Thus the report is considered complete when both results are on the floor.

Process Analysis

The analysis of the cycle time was done by collection of data on TAT for the departments of hematology and chemistry for the month of January 1992 (see Figure 5.8). A flowchart of the process is shown in Figure 5.9. The flowchart details the steps involved from collection of the specimen through reporting. In addition, an Ishikawa diagram relating the process components to the process delivery is shown in Figure 5.10. During this period of time, 44 spinal fluid specimens were analyzed. TAT data for both the chemistry and hematology departments were collected.

Data Summary

The table shows the average and standard deviations (s.d.) for the two departments. In addition, the longest of the two times was similarly analyzed.

	Chemistry	Hematology	Longest
Average	43.8 minutes	43.3 minutes	53.6 minutes
s.d.	24.4	26.5	25.8

Since there was no clear reason to continue analyzing the process in terms of the component departments, the process delivery was plotted in terms of the longest TAT. When this was done, one point appeared outside

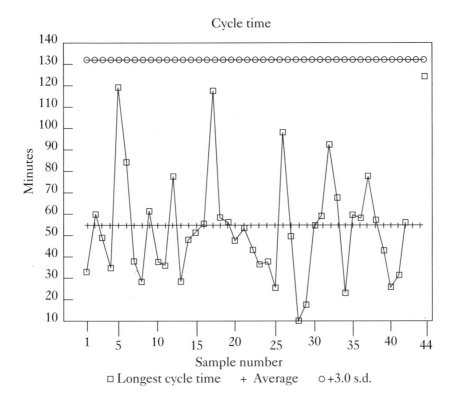

Figure 5.8: Spinal fluid cycle time, run chart.

of the normal process capability. This was a bloody tap, an example of special-cause variation. Consequently, the data were replotted to determine the system capability in absence of assignable cause. All points then appear within the 3 s.d. limits of the process performance.

Conclusions

The data suggest that all points, with the exception of one, represent routine process capability and, as such, can be assumed to be due to the normal variation associated with the process. This was confirmed by examination of the data for assignable cause. Some spinal fluids take longer than others when many cells are present. In the single case of the point outside 3 s.d., a very high red count of 1152 was seen. With regard to the points within the process capability, no correlation between cell count and TAT is evident.

In conclusion, the TAT of less than 90 minutes established by the medical director, while undoubtedly reasonable from the standpoint of medical necessity, is not consistent with the system capability. The natural tolerance limit (+3 s.d.) of this system is 131 minutes. Setting the upper

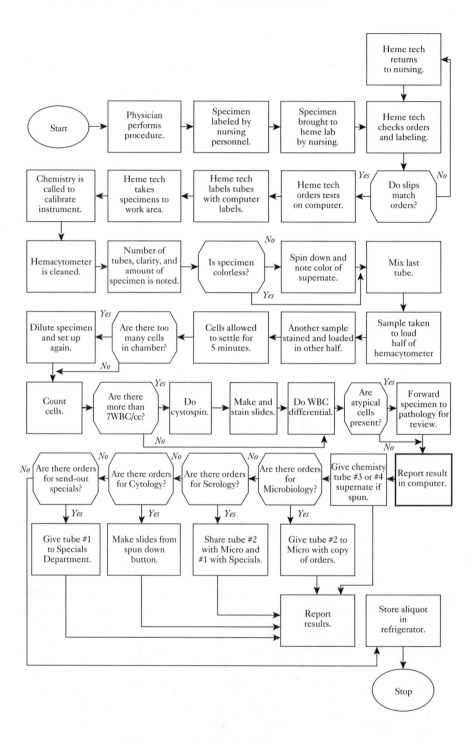

Figure 5.9: Spinal fluid cycle time, process flowchart.

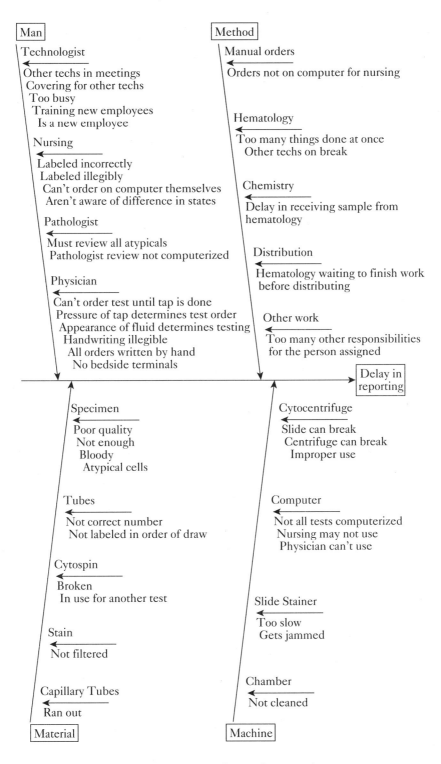

Figure 5.10: Spinal fluid cycle time, Ishikawa diagram.

specification limit at 90 minutes will result in a small percentage of the values falling naturally outside this specification, which is in keeping with observation.

This exercise allows management to focus on the system design and common variation to effect system improvement. Directing efforts at special- or assignable-cause variability will, in this particular case, be a waste of time. As a help in beginning the system analysis, the flowchart and the Ishikawa diagram may be used as starting points. As a parenthetical note, a histogram (not shown) of the January and February data (104 data points) indicates that the data are slightly skewed to the right. Standard techniques indicate that the conclusions reached are not affected by this finding.

NOTES

1. Process Management International, 7801 Bush Lake Road, Suite 360, Minneapolis, MN 55439-3315; 612-893-0313. PMI holds periodic seminars in which senior managers from Japanese TQC companies are invited presenters. These are an excellent opportunity for attendees to gain perspective on the Japanese quality movement as well as its adaptation to the West. The author wishes to thank Peter Malkovich, director of seminars, for permission to use the PMI version of the QC story.

2. John R. Hauser and Don Clausing, "The House of Quality," *Harvard Business Review* (May–June 1988): 63–73.

3. Vincent K. Omachonu, *Total Quality Productivity Management in Health Care Organizations* (Norcross, Ga.: Industrial Engineering and Management Press and ASQC Quality Press, 1991), 215.

6

Statistics

A modern TQM book isn't complete without a section on statistics. There are several reasons for this. First of all, Deming was a statistician, as was his mentor Shewhart, and they made a major contribution to Japanese TQC by showing how this difficult subject could be brought to the line level. Second, both in the United States and in Japan, statistical process control was an evolutionary step through which TQM moved, and much of the hard-core process improvement based on the Deming cycle uses statistical analysis as the basis for action. Lastly, the concept of process improvement—built around gaining statistical control through the SDCA cycle and eliminating assignable-cause variation, followed by process redesign to lower common-cause variation—is better understood with a good understanding of statistical theory.

Recall that some processes can be quantitated by the collection of data. The data come from a metric which is some measure of the process output or a dimension associated with the process output. Many processes cannot be quantitated due to the subjective nature of their results, however, but it is still important to think like a statistician: To view the product from the perspective of a statistician, taking into account the components of variation, the process capability, and the fitness of the process output as compared with customer-defined limits of its acceptability.

157

At this point it is important to understand a distinction regarding the two main types of statistical analysis that will be used. Fortunately, the clinical laboratory provides well-known examples of each type. The traditional statistics which are used to assign normal ranges entail collecting the assay data on a given analyte for many patients and doing an average and a standard deviation.

Similarly, if two instruments were running the same analysis to determine if they were similar, then a body of data run on both machines would be collected and compared. In both of these instances enumerative statistics is used. Enumerative statistics deals with the study of populations and is not concerned with the prior batch or the next batch from the process output.

TQM, however, is mainly concerned with analytical statistics, in which the focus of the statistical effort is on the ongoing process, and the intent is to derive information about subsequent performance from prior execution. This is similar to the use of control charts for run release where trends, shifts, and control limits are used to assess the ongoing utility of the analytical process.

At this juncture, I would like to comment on the selection of topics to be included here. Both SPC and conventional laboratory statistical use have been covered by experts in great detail elsewhere. The interested reader is referred to the references at the end of this chapter which are by no means exhaustive. I would, however, like to explore the relationship between the teachings inherent in SPC and those of clinical lab statistics.

To do this I must travel back into the gray mists of time to when there were hardly any computers. Actually, in the early 1970s computers had been around for quite some time, but the personal computer consisted of hand-held Texas Instrument models. There were also some early Wangs. Mostly there were mainframes which hardly anyone but large corporations could afford.

In those wild and primitive times, there were a few rugged individuals who were true pioneers in bringing statistics to the lab, and chief among these was Dr. James O. Westgard. Westgard wrote an early paper with Marion Hunt on method comparison. He simulated analytical data with built-in error of different sorts. Later he would write the article from which the "Westgard Rules" for run release were derived.

In addition, he published *A Shewhart Chart for Clinical Laboratory Use*, and therein lies the connection between the originator of SPC and the clinical lab. Just as Shewhart brought SPC to the Japanese through Deming, so Westgard brought it to the lab using the teachings of Shewhart and the axioms in Western Electric's *Statistical Quality Control Handbook*.

METHOD COMPARISON

There are many software packages available for statistics and graphical use that are quite easy to use. Statisticians suggest that the basic statistical equations behind any statistical analysis be known to users. Statisticians give examples of how people just shoved numbers into computer programs and got burned because of it. This is all true; hence my recommendation to become familiar with the material in the references at the end of this chapter. For the remainder of this chapter, however, I assume that you have access to one of these programs and that you can plug data in and get statistical analysis out.

It frequently occurs in the lab that two sets of data must be compared to see if there is any difference in the means or variances. This can occur when validating new instrumentation by comparing it with the old system, comparing a new assay technique with another one to verify that reference ranges are the same, or comparing two technologists to assure that training has been effective and that both operators are generating data with the same degree of reliability.

In these instances, several method comparisons may be used, one of which is the t-test. This is sometimes referred to as the Student t-test after the investigator who originally suggested its use, W. S. Gosset, who wrote under the pseudonym Student.

When using the t-test, the study can be set up so that the data are paired or unpaired. The paired design is intended to reduce the difference between the two runs by eliminating unforeseen variation due to such factors as different operators, different test days with potentially different environmental conditions, and so forth. To pair or not to pair, that is the question. Actually, it is not so much of a question as a factor to be accounted for when selecting the appropriate statistics. Pairing is one method of blocking out nuisance variables which is explored further in the section on design of experiments later in this chapter.

When plugging data into a t-test, the statistical program will generate several parameters, the bias (difference of the two mean values), standard deviation of the differences (SDd), and t.

Another way to compare two methods is to use linear regression. This generates least squares parameters m (slope), the y-intercept (b), and the standard error of the estimate (Sy). Two more parameters which are commonly used to compare methods are the Pearson product correlation coefficient (r), and the Fisher F test, which generates the parameter F from dividing the variances of the two processes.

Conventionally, the t statistic is used to determine if the two process means are the same or not, and the F statistic is used to determine if the variances may be considered equivalent. Juran cautions that if the two processes are found to be statistically different, then one may be reasonably confident that the processes will be different in practice. If the processes are found to be statistically the same, however, Juran cautions that upon further sampling they may indeed be found to be different. So, view this latter case with a certain amount of skepticism.

Westgard simulated three types of instrument error (constant, random, and proportional) and tabulated the effect of each of these on the conventional statistical parameters. His results are shown in Table 6.1.

Using the Pearson correlation coefficient (r) as an example, note that the two methods can have quite a large constant and/or proportional error, and the r value would still be 1.00 indicating perfect positive correlation. Further, Westgard and Hunt showed that the range of values also had an effect on r. For a constant random error of 10 mg/dl, the Pearson product was 0.764 for a range of 70 to 110 mg/dl, indicating a tolerable correlation. But for the same 10 mg/dl random error studied over the range 0–300 mg/dl, the Pearson product was 0.986 indicating much better correlation. In fact, the correlation is the same for both but the parameter misleads. Westgard and Hunt's article offers similar insight into the other parameters and emphasizes the wisdom of understanding the statistical parameters in depth. Westgard's findings are summarized in Figure 6.1.

Table 6.1: Summary of the sensitivity of conventional statistical parameters to different types of error.

| | *Type of error* | | |
Parameter	Random	Constant	Proportional
m	No	No	Yes
b	No	Yes	No
Sy	Yes	No	No
Bias	No	Yes	Yes
SDd	Yes	No	Yes
r	Yes	No	No

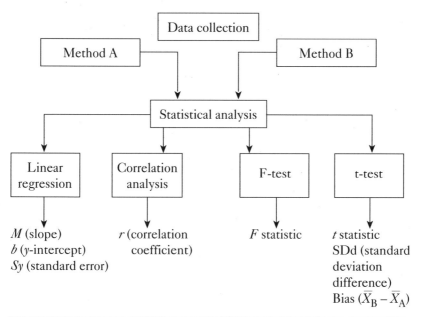

Figure 6.1 table:

		Proportional	Statistical
Random error	Constant error	error	test
Sy	b	m	$t: X_A = X_B$?
SDd	Bias	Bias	$F:$ sd$_A$ = sd$_B$?
r		SDd	

Figure 6.1: Statistical aspects of method comparison. The statistical comparison of two methods are shown using common statistical tools. The two methods can be two instruments, two different reagent systems on the same instrument, two different technologists, or the output of two different shifts as well as other methods for comparison. The parameters generated by these techniques are shown at the top. The bottom part shows the sensitivity of the generated statistical parameters to different types of error,* and the bottom right panel shows the use of the *t* and *F* statistics to delineate differences in bias and variance respectively.
*James O. Westgard and Marion Hunt, "Use and Interpretation of Common Statistical Tests in Method Comparison Studies," *Clinical Chemistry* 19 (1973), 49.

COMPONENT PROCESSES

Most processes can be broken down into components and that is why TQM offers several ways of analyzing processes in terms of their components such as root cause analysis, stratification, decision trees, and so on. The Japanese counsel to ask why five times is another way to access the root cause.

For instance, ask a process owner, "Why isn't the process working?"

"We don't know."

"Why don't you know?"

"We don't have the data."

"Why don't you have the data?"

"We asked MIS [management information services department] to modify the data collection program, but so far they haven't delivered."

Ask MIS, "Why no data collection software?"

"We sent our man to do it, but their system is always in use during our working hours."

Solution: Schedule an off-hours system change and validation.

From a statistical standpoint, it helps to know how some common statistical parameters behave when applied to process components. For instance, the laboratory can be viewed as a sequence of processes—A, B, and C, where A is the input to B, and C is the output of B. For instance, this would be where A = preanalytical, B = analytical, and C = postanalytical.

PROCESS VARIANCE

The variances, or squares of the standard deviations for processes, are additive. This helps to estimate the overall process variance when the component process variances either are known or can be estimated.

$$(\text{s.d.})^2_{\text{Total}} = (\text{s.d.})^2_A + (\text{s.d.})^2_B + (\text{s.d.})^2_C \qquad (6\text{-}1)$$

Recall that the CV is the standard deviation divided by the mean. If the component processes are varying around the same mean then,

$$(\text{CV})^2_{\text{Total}} = (\text{CV})^2_A + (\text{CV})^2_B + (\text{CV})^2_C \qquad (6\text{-}2)$$

The National Cholesterol Education Program used a similar approach in estimating the process capability in cholesterol measurement. By dividing the test reliability into preanalytical and analytical components, the lab standardization panel was able to arrive at a feasible target variance for overall laboratory test performance.

They postulated that if bias could be eliminated by calibrating to the same reference materials, then total analytical error would be random only, and it would be a combination of analytical and biological variability. Based on a prior study, the panel let analytical error (expressed as % CV) = 1.8 and biological variation = 2.8. The total variation, then, would be the square root of the sum of the squares of these two components or 3.32 percent.

RELIABILITY

The overall reliability of a three-part system $R(o)$ is the product of the individual reliabilities. Reliability is the probability of doing good.

$$R(o) = R(a) \times R(b) \times R(c) \tag{6-3}$$

Dr. Raymond Gambino recently remarked that the cytology error in Pap smears had three major components, the least of which was the reader error. In his view, the preanalytical components were most contributory. The largest, from the patient's health standpoint, was not having the test done at all, and the second was getting the specimen taken correctly.

PROCESS FOCUS IN THE HEALTH CARE INDUSTRY

Figure 6.2 shows the difference in focus of conventional versus health care concerns in relation to the utility of SPC. Health care concerns force a process designer to focus all of his or her efforts up front on assuring that the process performs flawlessly. Should this not be the case, and a rare event occur in which the process fails, then the Japanese recommend single-case boring. This is where these very rare instances are analyzed in detail in hopes of learning not statistical inference, but actual cause in order to modify the system to prevent future occurrence. This is done in airline crashes, for instance.

I shared this view with Kersi Munshi when he was a senior analyst at FPL. Munshi mentioned similar cases in the electrical power industry when working around high-tension wires. He said that the industry wouldn't want to record 20 workers falling off pylons before doing a statistical summary and presenting management with a process improvement opportunity. All of the design effort would again be focused on foolproofing the process up front, followed by single-case boring in the unlikely event of an accident.

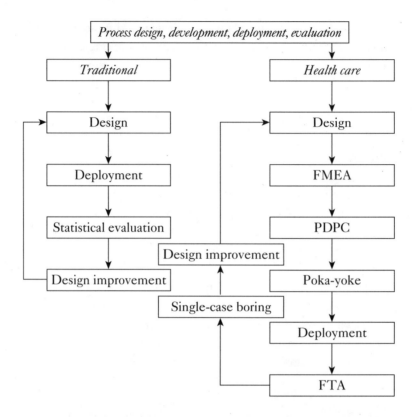

Figure 6.2: The health care focus and traditional TQM. The difference between traditional TQM process development and the process development in critical health care processes is shown by the traditional process being evaluated by statistical means following deployment. The health care process design focuses efforts on foolproofing prior to deployment and single-case evaluation afterward.

THE DIFFERENTIAL USE OF TRADITIONAL TQM METHODS AND POKA-YOKE

The clinical lab can be divided into the technical component and the service component. The technical part of lab testing is already under very good control. Techs are licensed and educated in the skills needed for their work. Specific on-the-job training is frequently provided by suppliers and equipment manufacturers who are experts in their products.

A recent example of federal regulations resulting in an exactly equivalent technical lab operation is the National Institute for Drug Abuse (NIDA).

This organization has issued regulations which resulted in toxicology labs performing tests in exactly identical ways to exactly identical standards. As a result, the quality of their technical services are indistinguishable. They can only compete in the areas of price, image, and service. This situation is only a matter of degree different from conventional clinical labs. The customer takes for granted the fact that the technical delivery will be perfect and responds only to service aspects of the lab.

Consequently, the lab image is directly linked with the service aspects which it offers. The lab service areas are the couriers, accessioning, technical service, communications, billing, and reporting. These service areas are common to many businesses and are amenable to process error reduction by the routine application of TQM principles. Where the service and technical areas merge is in phlebotomy. Clearly this is a preanalytical service which the lab may offer, but at the same time since it calls for absolute identification of the patient and the specimen, this area must be controlled as carefully as any other.

The technical areas of analysis and data transfer, however, show limiting returns from routine application of TQM. It only reduces the error to levels limited by the output of the human system itself. This isn't good enough in most instances. To further enhance human process capability, it is necessary to resort to the techniques of Shigeo Shingo, who called these methods poka-yoke. These can be mathematically modeled by the fractal set known as the Cantor Dust to represent the limiting error level of human system output.

Both Mandelbrot, who used the fractal set, and Shingo, who used other methods, reached the same conclusion. Only foolproofing could further lower operator error to levels low enough to be consistent with the acceptable error expected from health care systems.

Apparently foolproofing doesn't translate well into Japanese, and so poka-yoke is used. This is derived from the words *yokeru* (to avoid) and *poka* (inadvertent errors) to represent fail-safeing or mistake proofing. The idea is to design systems which have mechanical design forcing workers to do a process only one way. Whereas most of Shingo's examples are limited to manufacturing cases, the principle can be used in service process areas as well. Foolproofing and redundancy are special cases of Taguchi's robust process design. Here, processes are designed to be insensitive to external causes of special variation. In controlling, assessing, and improving the process delivery and capability of operations which are amenable to statistical review, however, the methods of sampling and the use of associated process control charts may be helpful.

SAMPLING

Clinical laboratorians are not accustomed to the concept of sampling and the traditional use of sampling in SPC. They do, however, sample when they run a control and measure a variable parameter which represents the process performance. Sampling does two things. First, it allows for an idea of how a process is running based on only looking at a representation of the process delivery. When testing the capabilities of Patriot missiles, for instance, good economics dictates choosing just the right minimum number of them to blow up to guarantee that a given lot will perform reliably. On a lesser scale, judicious control use is also good economics in the lab.

The second thing variables sampling does is also very important. The very act of sampling results in the samples being normally distributed. In the examples used, in method comparison, the statistical parameters require that the population under study be normally distributed, but, in fact, it is never really known with certainty that this is the case. Sampling assures this.

When the distribution is normal (gaussian), then the process capability index can be calculated. This is a qualitative indication of the process performance relative to specifications.

Sampling is a process whereby representative segments or portions of the whole are studied to gather an indication of the quality or condition of the entire lot of material. As will be discussed later, the FDA is shifting emphasis from sampling to process validation as a means to ensure quality of the process delivery. Sampling and validation are not, however, mutually exclusive. Properly done on a stable process, the sample can give a good indication of the lot or process capability. An understanding of these concepts is important in the lab since, at all steps of the analytical process, there are ways in which the progress can be reviewed, either completely or by sampling.

Juran says that there are three ways to evaluate a product or process. These are by

- No inspection
- Sampling
- 100-percent inspection

In the last case, for instance, 100-percent inspection might imply to the unwary that the outgoing report had been 100 percent checked by a supervisor and was free of error. This is, of course, not true since even 100-percent inspection, if done by human eyes, is subject to error. Consequently, in some critical operations, 200-, 300-, or even 400-percent inspection is the rule.

The major criterion for inspection is one of economics. For instance, for no inspection, the cost to the company is figured at $ NpA, where N = the number of items in the lot, p = the percent defective, and A = damage cost, which is the cost to replace or repair the defective item. Not accounted for is Deming's perspective that there is no way to estimate the damage done by creating a dissatisfied customer.

Since clinical lab results are frequently used for diagnosis or to indicate or modify treatment, the end user may be the patient whose health can be jeopardized by an erroneous result. In this case, since at least 100-percent inspection is used, the cost to the lab is $ NI where now N = the number of reports and I = the inspection cost for each report.

Sampling plans are designed to take advantage of economies when testing is destructive. In the lab area, however, at least in the reporting process, not much economic advantage can be taken. There are other areas in which sampling may be used to assess component process functions and to gather data for eventual process improvement.

RATIONAL SUBGROUPING

Rational subgrouping refers to collecting samples from preselected subgroups to yield additional insight into the process under study. For instance, if hematologists are doing manual diffs, the output of the department relative to standard check slides may be needed. The total error of the department can be assessed by repeating the check slides at random and combining the data. Rational subgrouping would direct that the data from subgroups consisting of individual technologists or different shifts be collected. Thus, if it turns out that any of the individuals are statistically different from the group output, then remediation can be directed to the individuals in a fashion that saves time and training resources. This is also in keeping with CLIA '88 which directs that individual performance be assessed periodically.

STATISTICAL PROCESS CONTROL

Statistical process control has been used since Walter A. Shewhart introduced it in the 1920s. Heavily used during World War II in this country, it was introduced to the Japanese by Deming in the 1950s. Some people view SPC as an evolutionary step through which management styles have progressed on their way to TQM. This evolution is reflected in Figure 6.3. The question mark indicates the uncertainty surrounding whether Japan will opt for some of the more humanistic values inherent in TQM or in Deming management.

SPC remains central to the evaluation of processes which generate enough data that statistical methods can be used for the evaluation and analysis of the system delivery. In fact, Deming says to cease reliance on final inspection, but he doesn't say to abandon it. His point is building in quality by process control before the product or service is in the hands of the final inspector, who is always the consumer.

SPC consists of various topics which focus on special- and common-cause variation, understanding and predicting it, and removing or minimizing it. Key to this undertaking is the control chart.

Control charts all have some commonality which include the centerline, frequently a mean value, and the upper and lower control limits, abbreviated by UCL and LCL. These are statistically derived from multiples of the standard deviation of the mean.

There are two major process characteristics from which control charts are generated. These are attributes and variables. Attributes consist of discrete occurrences, such as reactive/nonreactive, go/no go, acceptable/not acceptable, and the data are discontinuous, expressed as integers and multiples of these. Variables, on the other hand, have to do with measurements taken on a unit, such as radius, length, density, or concentration, (for example, glucose in mg/dl, or enzyme activity in IU/L). The data are continuous and can be expressed as fractions or decimals. Using a lot of steel bolts as an example, attribute sampling or classification would either list a bolt as acceptable or not acceptable based on its status overall. Attributes classification would pass or fail the bolt based on several sets of parameters including its length, diameter, thread pitch, and so on. Variables are more sensitive to process variability and provide more detailed information about the process.

The types of attribute control charts are as follows:

- *p* chart: percent defective in a sample
- *c* chart: number of defects in a sample
- *np* chart: number of defectives in a sample
- *u* chart: defects per unit in a sample

Plotting attributes, or conformance versus nonconformance, allows the usual control chart information to be retrieved such as scatter or variability of the process, whether or not the process delivery is smooth and under

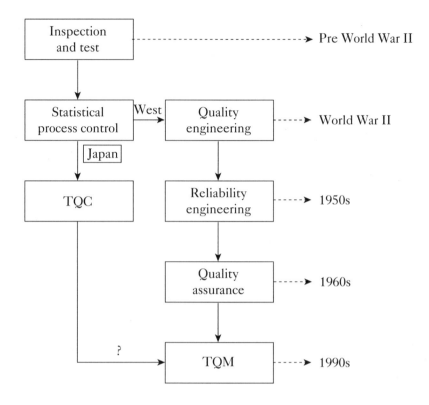

Figure 6.3: Evolution of quality management. The evolution of quality from a function which was the concern of a limited area or department, to the current role which is a management function with companywide responsibilities.

statistical control or whether or not the distribution indicated some assignable or special-cause variation, shifts, and trend. But attributes sampling doesn't get into the details of the process to shed light into the reasons for the process delivery shortcomings. In addition, attributes are discretely rather than continuously distributed, and, as a result, generally use statistics described by the Poisson, binomial, or other distribution functions which are applicable to discretely occurring processes. Figure 6.4 shows a flowchart for choosing the correct control chart based on the type of data collected.[1]

The most frequently used type of variable control charts is the $\bar{X}$–R chart where $\bar{X}$ is the average of measurements in a sample, and R is the range of measurements in a sample. These variables have a continuous distribution. In other words, glucose concentration doesn't come as one glucose, two glucoses, and so on. It has a distribution which varies continuously from zero to saturation. Upper limits encountered in the lab are mostly compatible

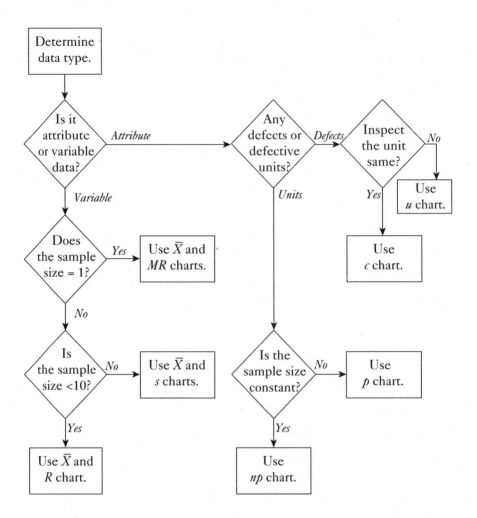

Figure 6.4: Determining which control chart to use. The relationship between attribute and variable data is shown with respect to the types of control charts suitable for plotting the different kinds of sampling.

with life, although in some emergency cases, not for long. These two variables are separately assessed and plotted independently. The sample averages are plotted around the grand average of all the samples, and a range, proportional to the standard deviation, is used to establish the upper and lower control limits. From these the process capability can be determined.

The process capability is an important indicator, because from it, one can see whether or not the required tolerances can be met. There is no sense in requiring more from the process than it is capable of delivering, and this technique will tell what it can do. The process capability is shown by the upper and lower tolerance limits, which are usually defined as three times the process standard deviation.

PROCESS CAPABILITY INDICES

Figure 6.5 shows one definition of the process capability index or C_p = USL – LSL/6 × s.d. where USL and LSL are the upper and lower specification limits. These are set externally by the customer. Process capability requires that variables sampling be used. This creates the normal distribution to which this definition of process capability applies. The ideal situation is where the process output has a mean centered about the specification target, and where the natural tolerance limits of the process are well within the specifications.

Another definition of the process capability index is given by C_{pk}. Figure 6.6 shows this defined as C_{pk} = [| process mean – nearer spec limit|]/ 3 s.d. In both cases, the higher the process capability index the better, since this means that the specs exceed the process capability by a wide margin and that the percent nonconforming will be small. U.S. industrial process capability in the 1970s measured in this fashion was about 0.8, whereas the Japanese minimum was 1.33.

SPC comprises a very rich and large body of knowledge, and the intention here is only to touch on some of the broader aspects of the subject. Before proceeding on, please note that the Levy–Jennings quality control charts that are widely used in the clinical lab are population charts and are different than what is discussed here. Nonetheless the Levy–Jennings plots of individual averages against a 2–3 s.d. range used for run release do share the commonly accepted indicators of out-of-control situations such as trends, shifts, and special-cause variability. These are more fully described for the sampling charts in Western Electric's *Statistical Quality Control Handbook*.

DESIGN AND ANALYSIS OF EXPERIMENTS

Design of experiments (DOE) is a formal discipline which enables individuals to intentionally change processes to explore the outcome of the intentional changes. Many times systems analysis is done retrospectively.

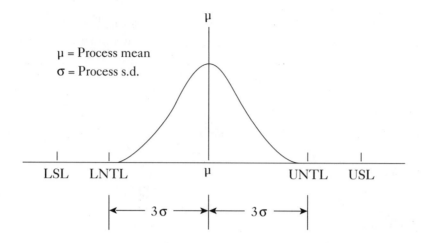

Figure 6.5: Process capability. A normal distribution showing the upper and lower natural tolerance limits (UNTL, LNTL) set at 3 s.d. from the mean. Note that the upper and lower specification limits (LSL, USL) are set by the customer and have nothing to do with the tolerance limits. One way of defining the process capability index is $C_p = (USL - LSL)/(6\sigma)$.

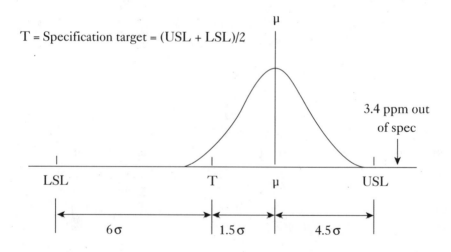

Figure 6.6: Process capability indices. Motorola has a six-sigma quality concept in which its target is no more than 3.4 defects per million. In this case the process capability index is defined as

$$C_{pk} = \frac{|\mu - USL|}{3\sigma}$$

Since Motorola defines its ideal process capability as $C_{pk} = 1.5$, reference to a Z table shows that the fraction out of spec is 0.00034 percent, or 3.4 ppm.

Whatever the system is generating in terms of outcome is studied, and using the PDCA cycle, change is initiated and the system is studied to observe the outcome. DOE is used to study systems in which there are many variables affecting outcome, and where it would be too time consuming to change each one and await the outcome. Analysis of experiments is inextricably linked to DOE, since one of the considerations in the experimental design is to incorporate enough attention to the design so that the data generated are capable of being analyzed, frequently by statistical means. This means that appropriate attention has been given to the design in terms of statistical requirements, such as randomization and repetition, so that the data, once analyzed, give insight into the process that couldn't be readily obtained by more conventional means.

The example given is the measurement of glucose in three different sites within a hospital. The objective is to assure that wherever the patient is within the hospital system, a glucose measurement will be the same within predetermined limits. Glucose (mg/dl) then becomes the response variable, the main variable under study.

Additional factors to consider are the time of day when the assay is done, the different personnel running the tests, the different instruments used, and the range (high/low) of testing. Since factors of interest are chosen, the design of experiment allows examination of these effects.

There are additional factors such as temperature, humidity, and operator stress levels. These are not studied. DOE allows experimenters to screen out these nuisance variables by a technique known as blocking. The influence of these factors is still there but the randomization method is such that they contribute equally to each set of measurements. Blocking is just the opposite of rational subgrouping in which variables are grouped so that their effects will be maximized and not confounded with other information. Experimental design B uses a technique known as chunk blocking. This results in intermediate sensitivity somewhere between confounding and rational subgrouping. By using chunk blocking, it is assumed that the time of day of the testing probably doesn't matter; that is, the instruments don't drift from morning calibration. Also one operator does all the testing so that no information will be gleaned about operator contribution to variability.

This clearly shows the effect of assumptions on the experimental design. Assumptions are routinely made to limit the scope of the experiments in keeping with resources and time factors. If the assumptions are wrong, however, the data will never reflect this. Thus, one of the major pitfalls of DOE is in overly parsimonious design which results in the generation of copious data leading to incorrect conclusions. Bad design yields bad results.

The following examples are illustrative only so that the reader may get a feeling for the utility of this technique. In practice, an expert statistical resource group, who will design more appropriate experiments tailored to the individual requirements of the study, should be used.

VALIDATION OF INTERLABORATORY ACCURACY AND PRECISION: EXPERIMENTAL DESIGN A

Objective: The objective of this experiment is to compare analytical accuracy and precision of analytical instruments in different physical locations. Each may impact diagnosis of the same patient at different times.

Background information

CLIA '88 mandates that instruments within a hospital setting, which can be used for the same analyte, are to be compared with each other. This way confidence can be had that the numbers generated from each instrument will result in the same diagnosis.

For instance, a patient may present to the emergency room in a coma. One of the causes may be diabetic coma caused by hypoglycemia. This may be initially diagnosed by a statlab instrument in the ER. The patient may be stabilized and sent to one of the critical care units where additional point-of-care (bedside) testing for glucose may be done. Subsequently, the main lab will be involved in routine monitoring during the patient's stay. All three testing instruments in different lab settings run at different times by different techs must yield the same results within the parameters set by clinical diagnostic needs. It is generally accepted that a true glucose value ±5 percent will fulfill this criteria.

To study these effects, both high (250 mg%) and low (70 mg%) glucose calibrators will be run as unknowns in the three locations. These will be called the high control (HC) and low control (LC). These represent the two main clinical presentations of hyper- and hypoglycemia. The values obtained in the labs will be compared against the known true values as an estimate of accuracy. In addition, repetition will be used to assess precision in each analytical setting.

In running this experiment it is assumed that the processes in each lab are stabilized; that is, the SDCA cycle has been addressed, all individuals are calibrating their instruments with the same control material, all individuals understand that blood for glucose measurement must be collected in stabilizers which prevent glucose degradation (glycolysis), and all techs are properly trained on their own particular instrumentation. To verify that this is true, the quality control data, which each lab collects as currently required by regulation, can be evaluated. The data must reflect that each analytical setting is currently running under statistical control and that no special cause effects are evident.

Experimental Variables
- Response variable—glucose value
- Measurement technique—Three instruments A, B, and C
- Factors under study
  —Instruments A, B, and C
  —Analyst within laboratory (two per lab)
  —Time when measurement made (directly after calibration = AC or before calibration = BC)
- Values within measurements window (two per tech per day)
- Background variables
  —Ambient conditions including temperature, humidity, and ER stress factors

See Figure 6.7 for a graphical schematic of this study.

Replication
The study cannot interrupt the normal lab testing schedule; however, once each shift the on-duty tech calibrates the instrumentation. In order to integrate this study smoothly, it is suggested that the high control and low control be run directly after the daily calibration, which will reflect optimum instrument condition, and just before the next shift calibration, which will reflect maximum instrument drift during the shift. Length of time is of little consequence so that replication can be done over eight days to collect a reasonable data accrual. Duplicate repetition of the daily measurement are made to assess precision.

Method of Randomization
A valid computer-generated randomization function is used.

Design Matrix

See Figure 6.7 for further explanation.

Control Level	Lab	Tech	Measurement
Low	ER	a	A.M. (×2), P.M. (×2)
		b	A.M. (×2), P.M. (×2)
	Unit	a	A.M. (×2), P.M. (×2)
		b	A.M. (×2), P.M. (×2)
	Main lab	a	A.M. (×2), P.M. (×2)
		b	A.M. (×2), P.M. (×2)
Low	ER		
	Unit	Etc.,	
	Main lab		
High	ER		Etc.,
	Unit		
	Main lab		
High	ER		Etc.
	Unit		
	Main lab		
High	ER		
	Unit		
	Main lab		
Low	ER		
	Unit		
	Main lab		
High	ER		
	Unit		
	Main lab		
Low	ER		
	Unit		
	Main lab		

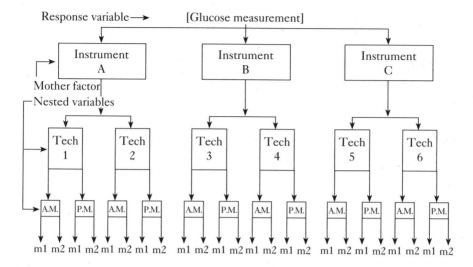

Figure 6.7: Validation of interlaboratory precision and accuracy—schematic of experimental design. The measurement of glucose at different locations within a hospital setting is a function of several variables which this experiment is designed to assess. The response variable, glucose concentration, is primarily a function of the three instruments which are located in the emergency room (A), the patient bedside (B), and the main lab (C). Nested within this mother variable are additional variables related to the analytical technologist in the department, and whether the measurement is made directly after the morning calibration (A.M.), or at the end of this shift when the instrument may have drifted (P.M.). Duplicate measurements are made at these times to assess precision (m1, m2).

Data Collection Forms

To be designed by the project leader.

Method of Statistical Analysis

The run chart, dot-frequency diagram, and estimate of components of variation are used.

Resource Considerations

The study uses data from eight days integrated with routine instrument calibration and two operators.

EXPERIMENTAL DESIGN B

This experimental design assumes a high degree of knowledge about the process. This way, rational subgrouping and appropriate chunk blocking can be used to combine and minimize nuisance variables. Thus, a paired t-test can be used to compare any instrument with the main lab instrument, which is now validated and maintained as the reference instrument.

This setup has a certain amount of validity inasmuch as the instrument controllers in the main lab are licensed and highly trained individuals with documented experience in analysis of body fluids. This is generally not the case for point-of-care analysts who may be given ad hoc training on foolproof instrumentation designed to be used by manufacturers in these environments.

First, the main lab instrument must be validated such that documentation of the instrument performance with time is well established. This can be done with an $\bar{X}$–R chart over a defined time period, and the instrument performance summarized. Secondly, a paired t-test can be run comparing the main lab instrument with others, one at a time. Then the comparisons are recorded and documented. The chunk blocking will now include time of day and instrument operator. Randomization will be used to record glucose readings at various times, and one main lab tech will be assigned to visit the various instruments to do the collection, thus obviating any performance variables attendant to local operators. This may not be strictly in accordance with intuition, but it is directly responsive to the regulatory language, which appears to tacitly assume that all variance is accorded to the instrument and is operator insensitive. By successively unblocking components of the paired analysis, the designer can assess, in a more leisurely fashion, the component effects of the contributions of nuisance variables.

Summary

The purpose of this chapter is to emphasize the highlights of TQM application of statistics. The reader is invited to consult the many excellent writings on these materials for a more in-depth presentation of the specific applications of statistical methodologies.

NOTE

1. Thanks to Jill Swift, Ph.D., University of Miami, Department of Engineering, for the use of this flowchart.

SUGGESTED READING

Amsden, Robert T., Howard E. Butler, and Davida M. Amsden. *SPC Simplified: Practical Steps to Quality*. White Plains, N.Y.: Quality Resources, 1989.

Burr, Irving W. *Statistical Quality Control Methods*. New York: Marcel Dekker, 1976.

Corporate Quality Education and Training Center. *Continuing Process Control and Process Capability Improvement*. Dearborn, Mich.: Ford Motor Company, 1987.

Duncan, Acheson J. *Quality Control and Industrial Statistics*. 5th ed. Homewood, Ill.: Richard D. Irwin, 1986.

Harry, M. J. *The Nature of Six-Sigma Quality*. Schaumburg, Ill.: Motorola University Press, 1987.

Moen, Ronald D., Thomas W. Nolan, and Lloyd P. Provost. *Improving Quality Through Planned Experimentation*. New York: McGraw-Hill, 1991.

Western Electric Company. *Statistical Quality Control Handbook*. Indianapolis, Ind.: AT&T Technologies, 1956. (11th printing, 1985).

Westgard, James O., Robert W. Burnett. "Reassment of Precision Requirements for Analytical Methods." *Clinical Chemistry* 36 (1990): 1004.

Westgard, James O., Robert W. Burnett, and George N. Bowers. "Quality Management Science in Clinical Chemistry: A Dynamic Framework for Continuous Improvement in Quality." *Clinical Chemistry* 36 (1990): 1712–1716.

Westgard, James O., and Marion Hunt. "Use and Interpretation of Common Statistical Tests in Method Comparison Studies." *Clinical Chemistry* 19 (1973): 49–57.

Yost, Gerald, M.D., Ph.D. "The Hybrid Laboratory." *Medical Laboratory Observer* 24 (September 1992 supplement): 1.

7

Implementing TQM

The object in launching TQM into a conventional business setting is aimed at changing the company culture from the old paradigm to the new. When Kano and the Japanese consultants did this at FPL they admitted that their techniques were aimed at breaking the back of the old culture. Their strategy was to ruthlessly drive out any allegiance to the established system prior to installing TQC.

Implementing TQM can best be done in conjunction with outside consulting groups that are experienced in TQM deployment. If you elect to effect a rapid paradigm shift, don't try it with internal people alone. Too many egos will be bruised in the process, and it will simply instill a resentment for the new system that is exactly opposite the desired effect. In any event, it is considered too brutal for western tastes, and many deployment techniques are based on acknowledging the existing system and effecting a gradual change to the new paradigm. This is in keeping with the spirit of TQM as a process of gradual and continual improvement. It also keeps morale high. Don't, however, view TQM as an add-on to the existing culture. The old paradigm must be replaced with the new one. TQM must be totally deployed in a logical, intelligent, consistent fashion which eventually replaces the old system entirely.

Figure 7.1 shows the quality diamond which portrays the three major components of TQM—the voices of the business, the customer, and the employee. These must be integrated into the TQM process in order to establish the rational short-term goals for the company. The overriding benefits of TQM come not so much from people doing their jobs better, but from top management changing policy from things like performance salary review and MBO to the new TQM philosophies and teachings.

Another goal in the initial stages is to get people away from output, outcome, goal, and results orientation. Instead, they should think of the business as a system composed of different ongoing processes some of which they are involved in. This shift in mind-set should help people realize that they may interact with other ongoing processes either as users or suppliers.

Another goal in the early stages of TQM implementation is to integrate the voice of the customer with the voice of the business. This requires identification of the major customers in the lab operation. These are the consumers, both patients and physicians, and internal and external customers. These are also the regulatory agencies that expect the lab to perform in keeping with their regulations, and the people who make up the laboratory operation. In effect then, there are three major customer groups—the employees, the regulators, and the consumers of the lab output.

Figure 7.2 shows the top management objectives as defined in the company business plan and how to deploy these downward through hoshin kanri or management by policy. This method works best for a community of workers who are already well trained in the basics of TQM and quality in daily work. It is a reasonable way to start with the lab community. The fatal flaw in this deployment is that if the workers don't know TQM, then the deployment will flounder at the level of line management on down.

A second way to start is by training the line management and workers in TQM in daily work. There is a lot to be gained from this, but the efforts may become fragmented and disorganized due to a lack of focus provided by understanding management aims. Process improvement groups, while showing short-term gains in local process improvement, may eventually become parochial in their efforts and link poorly to the company and customer goals. This is analogous to the same car and the same driver, just more people in the backseat. This is also typical of TQM efforts in companies with minimal senior management involvement.

While beginning the management by policy organization, the TQM deployment must incorporate simultaneous training of line managers (the people who will eventually be the process owners) and workers. Imai says

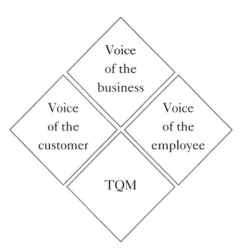

Figure 7.1: The quality diamond. This represents the three components of TQM. The voices of the business, the customer, and the employee are integrated into the ongoing TQM effort. The components are continually changing and must be continually accessed to maintain the integrated system.

that TQC begins and ends with training. The education of upper-level management, in addition to incorporating the basic curricula of the line people, must also include upper-level TQM business philosophy including Deming's theory of profound knowledge, and the 14 points.

Just as it is imperative to have top-level endorsement of the TQM effort in order for it to succeed, it is equally important to have top-level understanding of all facets of TQM. The introductory educational efforts must be tailored to executive tastes, and in this instance, it is sometimes best to encourage outside presenters. This way the executives aren't forced to listen to people who may be considered subordinates.

Top-level executives need to know this material not only to be able to provide guidance for developments arising from line-level process improvement, but they also need to chart a company course which is responsive to the voice of the customer and which provides opportunity and encouragement to innovation and breakthrough. To do this requires not just the skills of TQM learned by rote, but also an internalizing—a converting of knowledge into a plan which derives its motivation from internal resources and beliefs, not from external pressures and expectations. For TQM to succeed, senior management must be visibly involved in deployment and support of the effort.

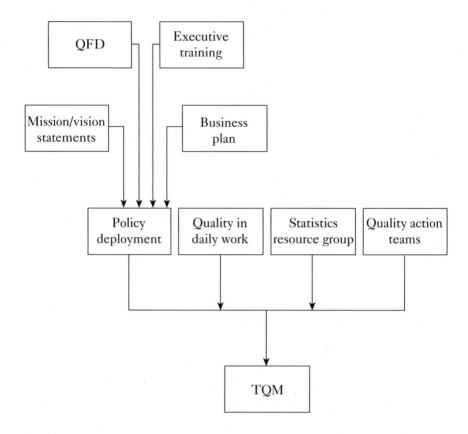

Figure 7.2: TQM deployment. One way of viewing the component processes of TQM. This must be skillfully blended with the other components of TQM through cross-functional management.

In training the trainers and developing companywide course curricula, it is important to avoid cascading. This is where one person trains 10 others, and each of these 10 then train 10 more, and so on. This is like the game of telephone where the message at the distal end is garbled in the transmission. Clearly one person can't train a thousand others in a timely way. The first group will grow impatient and forget the message by the time the last group internalizes the teachings. So there must be many trainers; but to keep uniformity throughout the business, it is important to rely on formal training curricula and video and written manuals of procedures.

The next step is identifying and standardizing processes and process owners within departments. It cannot be overemphasized that the TQM process improvement techniques will work just as well at standardizing a bad process as they will a good one. Therefore, it is important to identify a process and flowchart the best practice method. For instance, in transporting specimens from accessioning to the work areas, on close examination, there may currently be 10 ways to do this depending on who is in that day, what shift it is being done on, and so forth. The first pass at process improvement is to get all of the process owners together for this operation, flowchart the different ways it is being done, agree on the best practice method, and standardize this in actual operation. Make everyone do it the same way. Then analyze and collect data on the standardized process and improve on that.

THE ROLE OF MIDDLE MANAGEMENT

Middle management has had a hard time in U.S. business lately. Companies who are bent on streamlining their operations generally attack and lay off many people who they believe they can do without. Frequently their suspicions are justified after the layoffs by finding out that, in fact, the company may run as well or even better without the middle managers who got axed.

Deming, in his earlier attacks on western business practices, also let middle managers have it, in referring to them as buffers who were responsible for insulating upper management from the problems and needs of the work force. All of this must be reviewed in light of the role of middle managers in a TQM business society. It not only needs review, but the picture of the middle managers as communication buffers, or supernumeraries, is totally out of keeping with their role under TQM. Under TQM, the middle managers are one of the principle elements in making certain TQM works.

Under the old MBO system, middle managers frequently became superfluous, because the objectives they established were reflections of their own training and experience. Although these differed from department to department, they ended up being essentially self-serving rather than serving the business. It was no wonder then, that on firing one of the middle managers, the process of getting things done from the top suddenly became easier. The middle manager's personal goals were gone and replaced by upper management goals. Thus, workers were responding directly to what the business leaders wanted done.

The problem with this in the long run is that the executive group should be concentrating on long-term goals rather than the daily work goals in order for the company to progress and stay competitive. Thus, it should be obvious that the role of the middle managers is to execute the upper-level strategies and to assist in getting feedback from the work force back up to upper management.

This is depicted in Figure 7.3. Here it is shown that middle managers must act as facilitators of information flow in both directions. To do this, it is helpful to think of the executives and the workers as speaking different languages, with the middle managers responsible for translation. Juran calls this being bilingual. When this is the case, the middle managers need to be fluent in both languages to perform responsibly in this role.

In this fashion, both criticisms of middle management, acting as a buffer and effecting personal goals instead of upper management goals, are dispelled. In fact, the picture is reversed, and the middle managers become indispensable to an authentic TQM effort. They execute the rational goals of the executive and upper management group. They also identify strengths and recognize opportunities for improvement in the work force and help convey these to upper management levels for appropriate action.

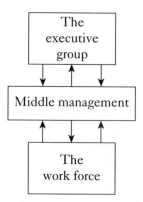

Figure 7.3: Middle management's role in TQM. Middle management assumes a key role under TQM. The middle managers must speak the language of the executive group as well as that of the work force. The middle managers are responsible for the downward deployment of management by policy (hoshin kanri), as well as the upward response of the work force to the established policies.

THE ROLE OF UPPER MANAGEMENT
AND THE EXECUTIVE GROUP

Leon Uris in *Trinity*, his book about Ireland, sums up the system there by saying that ". . . in Ireland there is no future, only the past happening over and over." Similarly, the executives of western companies continue to promulgate management practices which will eventually become extinct under the pressures from world competition springing principally from Japanese TQC. This extinction can come about in two ways. One is from the company itself vanishing in the unequal contest against TQC companies, and the other is by the executive group adopting the new ways and competing successfully in the new world market.

The initial thrust of TQM is to change the executive perspective from the traditional pattern to one nurtured in the intellectual gardens of TQM. The major benefits to the company come from this reorientation and not from changes at lower levels. Gitlow refers to this as the "paradigm shift" stemming from executive reorientation followed by introduction of the new methods and conceptions throughout the company by management by policy.

To effect this reorientation, Figure 7.4 illustrates the concentration of learning techniques focused on the executive group which must be complete prior to effective TQM implementation. Of the suggestions there, the only one needing additional explanation is listening to other TQM executives speak on their successes. Under the profound knowledge system, this can result in adopting a new method without understanding the basics, and this can lead to major problems, or in Deming's words, "a disaster." The reason a TQM ideology will work at another company is primarily an understanding of all the issues by the executive group at that company. Adopting another company's techniques without the in-depth understanding of how and why they work is a tempting shortcut, but the borrowed techniques may not work where you are.

THE ROLE OF THE WORKER

Just as the executives and middle managers have specific responsibilities under TQM, so do the workers. Their first responsibility is, as always, to do their job. This is sometimes overlooked in the promise of a rosier future under TQM, but it remains basic to the work force. This is

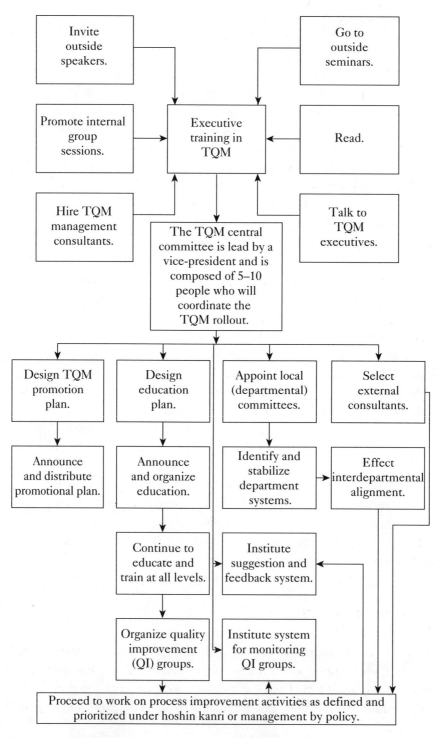

Figure 7.4: Introduction and implementation of TQM.

not asking anything more of the workers than is asked of the managers or the executives, but if the executives and managers understand TQM and are using it, then the job of the workers becomes easier.

The workers' job is easier because management is now accepting responsibility for improper process design, whereas in the past, management would often blame workers for common-cause problems. These were problems which were not under the workers' control and not within the workers' ability to fix. So in this sense, the work becomes more straightforward inasmuch the operators are now responsible for things over which they have control. In addition, process ownership is more clearly defined so that the individuals who are responsible for making certain the process is running smoothly and is steadily improving are clearly known.

Workers are also involved in something quite new, and that is in their participatory role in decision making and process improvement. This is done by three systems—the process improvement group, the quality circle, and the suggestion program. Additionally, workers may be involved in periodic executive reviews.

THE ROLE OF THE INDIVIDUAL

The Japanese believe that TQM begins with individuals and that the teachings of Deming should be applied to improve the personal life of individuals. By using TQM in one's personal life, the Japanese feel that the energy derived from the internal commitment to this effort will result in a more stress-free and vigorous approach to both the office and the home.

Personal growth in the quality arena can be made through active membership in the American Society for Quality Control (ASQC). ASQC is one of the fastest growing professional societies in the United States and currently has over 100,000 members. The membership increase of 25,000 in 1990 to over 80,000 put ASQC in the top 3 percent of U.S. professional societies in terms of growth.

Many workers are trained and educated in specialties which traditionally have had nothing specifically to do with quality. For these folks the question is where to go for credentialing and training. ASQC is a good first stop because its rapid growth reflects a growing national awareness of the organization's key role in quality. In addition, ASQC has the credentialing programs, and ASQC membership puts the member on mailing lists from many quality areas.

The credentialing exams are open only to people with prior background in quality, but the quality areas are more openly defined in terms of the TQM philosophy of responsibilities extending to all areas. Still, the certified quality engineer (CQE) requires eight years appropriate work experience past the bachelor's degree. Even so, only about 30 percent of applicants pass the CQE exam on first try. It is not something that can be readily learned from traditional work-related experience.

Reviewing for the CQE requires some knowledge of Deming and particularly Juran. The exam is weighted heavily on statistics, and knowledge of SPC is critical. The remainder references historical material as well as more modern material such as the systems approach to process improvement. There is nothing in the review that is actually contrary to Deming management, and there is much that sets the novitiate on the right path to both the systems and the statistical view. As a final note, the test questions were recently modified to include more modern material in the CQE exam.

Finally, American universities are just now beginning to offer courses which address TQM areas in a comprehensive fashion. None of them to date has the countrywide recognition which the CQE does. In addition, familiarity with the CQE exam will provide the pilgrim with exposure to the basic body of knowledge that one needs to explore and evaluate the recently emerging academic programs.

In addition, the laboratory professional associations are beginning to exhibit a more acute awareness of the role TQM is to play in their profession and are making materials available to their membership. This is a state of affairs which is certainly bound to continue apace.

Many individuals when first exposed to TQM as a management technique logically react by saying, "But I don't manage anything." The point to emphasize is that people at all levels manage things all the time, not only on their job, but away from it as well. They manage to get up in the morning, clean up, dress up, and get to work. At work they may start by organizing their day, arranging their work area, and doing other job-related operations. These are managed component processes of the overall company work effort. The better employees do them, the better for the company.

In addition, TQM recognizes that employees—line workers—have a closer perspective on their jobs than anyone else. It is therefore necessary that employees be trained well, not only about their jobs, but also about TQM. This way they know how to effectively promote process improvement and can get it done effectively within the company management framework. For employees to have good ideas, and no way to pass them on to upper management, and no reason to do so, simply squelches this very important facet of TQM. The work environment must foster employees' involvement in the improvement of aspects of their own jobs, and this is done by training, encouragement, a mechanism for transfer, and regard and recognition for all employees' efforts.

THE VISION AND MISSION STATEMENTS

The company's mission and vision statements are the capstone of the TQM process, because it is these discernments which are integrated into the company operational plan through hoshin kanri. This means literally target and means (hoshin) control (kanri). Its western name is management by policy. Management by objective integrates local managerial goals with subordinates. In contrast, management by policy integrates where the company is and where it wants to go with each and every department, division, and individual. Inasmuch as these two high-level policy statements are so important to the overall activity, their details are best well understood.

The vision statement is the company's long-term goal and represents where the executive group would like to see the company positioned from three to 10 years in the future. The statement offers no means of getting there, it isn't a strategy statement, and it is not a financial statement. No financial goals are incorporated in it. The statement is generally brief, but gives all employees a target on which to set their sights—a long-term goal to pursue.

The mission statement is a statement of what the company is in business to do currently. There are no futuristic overtones to it—the focus is on today, not tomorrow. Still, it should be as profound as possible without being overly pompous.[1,2] Possible pitfalls in the formation and use of the mission statement include behaving like the mission statement is a fait accompli, or thinking that the mission statement is cast in stone.

Many executives, upon forming the mission statement, proceed to forget about it as if the statement itself was the goal. This is old-paradigm thinking—thinking that slogans get the job done. Similarly, believing that the mission statement is cast in stone can also be a problem. As long as the business continues to do what it always has, then the mission statement can stay put; but the vision statement should change as the market changes. Both these statements can be judiciously changed to keep the company on the course deemed most appropriate by senior management.

VALUES AND BELIEFS

Values and beliefs are the boundaries on the road which the corporate culture travels on its way to the goals set out by the vision and mission statements. Values and beliefs form the pattern within which the individuals of the corporation operate. Company values come from an in-depth understanding of human nature, both from the standpoint of the individuals who make up the company payroll and from the standpoint of the people who are customers, suppliers, and vendors with whom the company does business.

The company's values and beliefs are best gleaned from professionals in the domain of psychology, sociology, and cultural anthropology. In some businesses this acumen may be found in the human resources (HR) department. While HR are traditionally thought to focus inward on the company employees, in a TQM sense, HR also focus outward to provide insight into general strategies which may be used to relate to people in any business setting. This is separate from the marketing perspective which concentrates on what people may buy for what price and when. In setting values and beliefs, do not hesitate to get outside counsel on these issues. Most helpful will be experts brought in from local academic and professional institutions to provide insight and provoke thought. When the values and beliefs have been established they should be published and made widely known to the work force.

As a parenthetical note, the August 1, 1990 issue of *Employment Review* credits Whitt Collins, president of West Coast Employer's Association of Tampa, Florida with the following study. Given 10 employee needs, the owners, managers, and supervisors ranked the needs in the left column as they thought the employees would rank them. The actual ranking done by the employees is in the right-hand column. The difference shows the disparity in thinking between the management perspective of what is important and the employees' view of what is most meaningful to them.

Owner/Manager/Supervisor Ranking

1. Higher wages
2. Job security
3. Promotion and growth
4. Better working conditions
5. Interesting work
6. Loyalty of fellow workers

Employee Ranking

1. Full appreciation for a well done job
2. Being included in office projects
3. Understanding and help on the job, including help with personal problems

7. Tactful discipline

8. Full appreciation of
   a job well done

9. Understanding and help
   on the job, including
   help with personal problems

10. Being included in office projects

4. Job security

5. Higher wages

6. Interesting work

7. Promotion and growth

8. Loyalty of fellow workers

9. Better working conditions.

10. Tactful discipline

INTEGRATING THE COMPANY'S MISSION
AND VISION WITH THE BUSINESS

Figure 7.5 shows how the mission and vision statements are blended with the voices of the customer, employee, and business to create prioritized outputs which are deployed throughout the company. These are used for setting rational goals for each department, division, and individual within these business segments.

Figure 7.6 shows a quality council, which is an operational group preferably headed by the company president. It is responsible for translating the mission statement into long-term operational goals. These are goals which are real in the sense that they can be further translated into lower level actions. The quality council may use the affinity diagram as a way to organize the output of its brainstorming sessions. The major headings of the affinity diagram would be the long-term goals upon which the company should take its direction. It is key that this council be headed by the most senior of executives, since without this insight the translation suffers and becomes distorted.

The enterprise at this point is broken into at least two activities. In the lab, or any regulated business, it may be broken down into several other segments. Directors and department heads may be utilized at this point for input regarding their specialties. The two major headings are the voice of the business, and the voice of the customer.

At this level, the voice of the customer is the consumer. This may be accessed through quality function deployment, and the customer needs identified. In any regulated business, however, there are at least two other customers whose voice must be identified. These are the regulators and the employees. The regulatory requirements of OSHA, FDA, HCFA, Nuclear Regulatory Commission (NRC), Enviromental Protection Agency (EPA), Department of Enviromental Regulation and Management (DERM), CLIA '88, Medicare, and state and local organizations must all be heard and put into

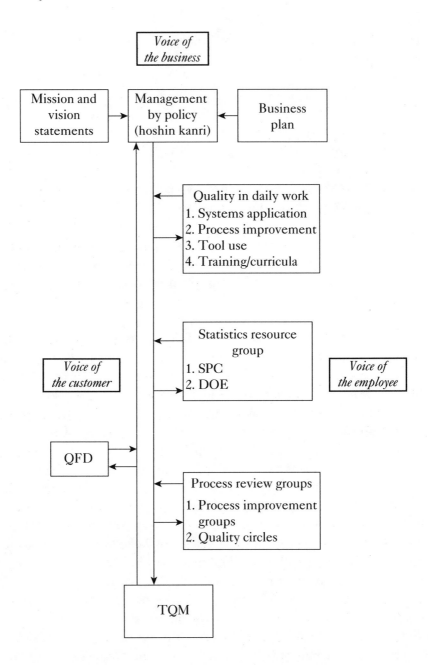

Figure 7.5: Integrating the voices of the customer, the employee, and the business with TQM. Linking TQM with the customer's requirements, the business's objectives, and the employee's needs and suggestions is key to making TQM work. The business system must provide for a clear and easily understood chain of command and information distribution. The system must also provide for a timely and controlled response to the information flow as needs are identified and prioritized for action.

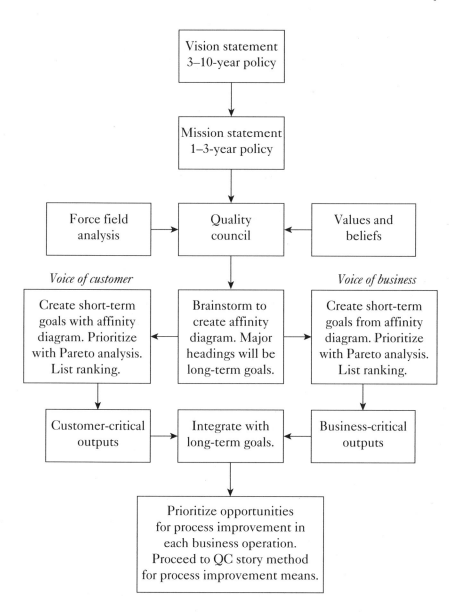

Figure 7.6: Hoshin kanri or management by policy. The deployment of TQM consistent with management by policy.

the matrix representing the customer's various voices. These are also quite high concerns, since to ignore any of the regulations, or to establish them at too low a priority, can be disastrous to the business. Similarly with the voice of the employee, the concerns which make the workplace a delight to work in must be addressed and brought to the table for prioritization.

The voice of the business links the mission statement to management by policy. At this point, the short-term goals are generated and these are prioritized by Pareto analysis for the voice of the business and also for the voice of the various customers. This prioritization generates critical outputs which are weighted short-term goals.

These goals, with their respective weights, are then linked through a matrix diagram which establishes the relationship (or lack of a relationship) between what the business priorities currently are and what the customer priorities currently are. This link is, of course, crucial to determine the order in which subsequent process improvement is generated. The entire focus is to set goals which are deemed rational, because they relate what the business can do with what the customers want. The goals are also prioritized so that the finite company resources can be concentrated on the areas which have been identified as being the most important.

I have tried to make this prologue as clear as possible, but at the same time I hope that it didn't appear simple, because these are not easy concepts. To do this for the first time successfully would be some sort of business miracle. This doesn't mean that you can't try, but I would suggest getting outside professional help at this point to facilitate your way through the process. What the preceding explanation should make clear is what you will need help in doing. When you seek counsel at least you will know what it is for. I was once told that to deal successfully with attorneys you had to know the aspects of law relating to your business better than they did. Similarly, with TQM deployment, you have to know what help to ask for before you can ask for the help you need.

INTEGRATING MANAGEMENT BY POLICY
WITH DAILY WORK AND IMPROVEMENT TEAMS

At this point in TQM deployment, the second of the three major components of TQM is brought to bear. This is the quality in daily work (QIDW) group. This group's function is to respond to the short- and medium-term goals as set forth by management by policy and translate these into process improvement opportunities. Usually, the QIDW group is composed of department managers and supervisors. These are the process owners who can translate what the executive level has prioritized into regional priorities for improvement. They are the meat in the sandwich portrayed in Figure 7.3.

The third major component of TQM, following management by policy and the QIDW group, are the teams. These are the process improvement groups, the quality action teams, the task teams, and the quality circles. These groups are formed of individuals at the line level who are most acquainted with the actual job processes which they perform. Most of these will be formed from groups within a department, although there will be ample opportunity to clean up lines of process input and output between departments. In this case the groups are called cross-functional in that they are now composed of people from different departments all focusing on a single opportunity.

The Japanese believe that a consumer views a product from three aspects—quality, cost, and scheduling. This translates to whether or not the company can deliver the goods or services that I want, at a reasonable cost, and when I want it. Consequently, the charter of the cross-functional teams is to integrate these broad functional areas backward into the company and across all departments and business functional units. Recently, safety has been added as a fourth cross-functional issue, but others feel that the quality area is broad enough to include this concern.

Figure 7.7 shows the relationship of the three components of TQM—policy deployment, QIDW, and quality improvement teams. This triangle is modified slightly from the triangle designed by the Union of Japanese Scientists and Engineers. The diagonal line cuts across the layers

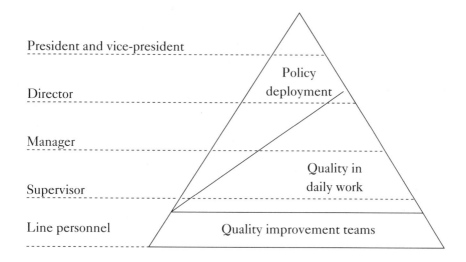

Figure 7.7: The TQM triangle. This triangle, from the Union of Japanese Scientists and Engineers (JUSE), represents the involvement of the various personnel levels in the three primary functions of TQM deployment. These are hoshin kanri (management by policy), quality in daily work, and quality teams. All are involved in the process of kaizen or continual improvement.

of management and shows the relative proportion of time, or the proportion of effort, the various levels commit to the three TQM elements. The executive and senior management group focuses primarily on management by policy, and translating the vision and mission statements to medium- and short-term company goals. The short-term goals are rational goals derived from integrating customer, employee, and business perspectives.

The QIDW group of the managers and supervisors and the line personnel participate to a lesser extent in policy deployment. Instead, the focus of the managers becomes one of prioritizing and aligning their own short-term goals with the senior management goals. This is done in Japanese TQC by a means called *catchball*. This is a technique, reflecting the word itself, in which the ideas of the executive group and the ideas of the directors are tossed back and forth to reach a meaningful deployment of the senior management goals at the line level. Various TQM planning tools are used to help expedite this process. The effort is conducted in such a way as to let the directors and supervisors, the process owners who are intimately acquainted with their process capabilities, buy in to the best way of effecting this translation. These people are key to getting this done. The deployment at this stage also must make room for creativity. Meaningless compromises must be avoided, but at the same time so must mindless compliance. This is a task in which skill and experience are helpful. Once again, I suggest a professional facilitator to help make this process go effectively. Once done, the responsibility of the QIDW group is to focus on daily processes which the business does in a routine fashion, but which are now prioritized for action related to their improvement.

The next functional group is the line-level teams. Seen from the triangle, these are formed primarily of people who have the keenest view of the line processes. These are the people who actually do the daily work and, as a result, are most able to reflect on what can best be done to improve the things which make line work easy and effective. There are three basic types of teams—the quality circle, the cross-functional task team, and the intradepartmental task team.

The quality circles are usually formed from a group within a department. This group, consisting of three to five people, exists in perpetuity and chooses tasks which relate to stabilizing and improving processes within the department. Frequently, quality circles take descriptive names, not unlike teams elsewhere from bowlers to flight crews. The quality circles are most similar to the intradepartmental task teams. These process improvement groups also operate within the department, but are formed to address a particular task which has been identified by prioritization as needing prompt attention. While the quality circle continues for as long as the group wants to continue it, the task team is dissolved when the process issue has been resolved.

The interdepartmental or cross-functional task team is a group formed from members of different departments who meet to address issues which extend across departmental boundaries. This group is usually headed by a manager or supervisor who facilitates the group in reaching process improvement for the cross-functional opportunity. Again, this group disbands after achieving improvement in keeping with cost and, as in the other group cases, documents its process improvement method.

THE SEQUENCE OF TQM DEPLOYMENT

Figure 7.8 is a Gantt chart for deploying TQM consistent with the details just reviewed. The key to making TQM deployment work is the concept of just-in-time training. The training of the individuals at each step and level must be done in such a fashion that there is no delay between their training and their ability to put the training to practical use. Think of the deployment curve as being a continuous trajectory in which the momentum is derived from a carefully thought-out sequence of training events.

In Figure 7.8, the deployment begins with executive management training in courses which include the philosophy and history of TQM, the management and QC tools, systems theory and statistics, and team dynamics. This series of topics, since they are key to TQM overall, will be repeated at different levels with a different emphasis. For the executive group, a focus on the philosophy, principles, and systems theory is a must in order for it to effectively create the mission and vision statements in keeping with TQM, and then link these to the voice of the business through management by policy. In addition the executives need to form a quality council to coordinate the overall TQM effort.

The quality council must then establish the feedback system for direct employee input, the statistics resource group, and the QIDW group. These groups must also be trained and be made ready for their subsequent roles. The quality council can then begin to work with the QIDW group on prioritizing the medium- and short-term goals which senior management sees as critical for ensuing action at the departmental level.

A word on statistics at this point. A theme which I have woven throughout this book is the difference between the lab industry and more general consumer industries for which TQM was initially designed. I have

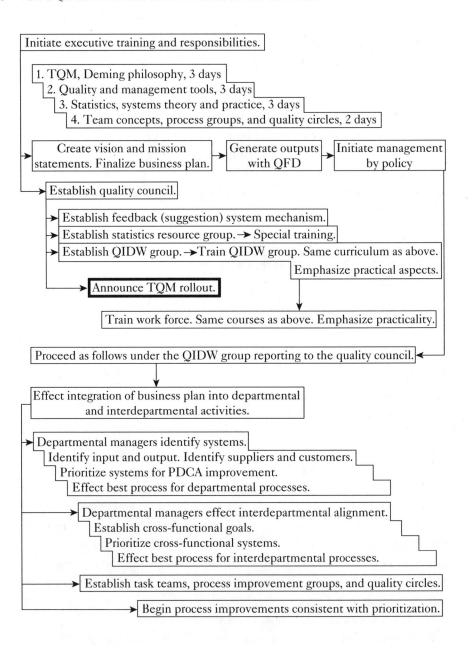

Figure 7.8: TQM implementation schedule. A schedule for implementing TQM is shown in Gantt chart form. Tasks shown with a parallel left border may be implemented simultaneously. Tasks with a staggered left border are sequential. The schedule begins with the executive training and ends with the first process improvements. The purpose of this schedule is to permit just-in-time training for all groups so that forward momentum is not lost by false starts. Each group knows when it will be trained in what subjects and what the object of the training is. Each step of the schedule shows the responsibilities of each group.

focused on designing systems which have a low probability of failure irrespective of the operators who perform the steps within the systems. Industry has adopted this strategy in many critical areas in which redundancy or foolproofing are also used. Wherever the emphasis, the need to think like a statistician in term of process design and process reliability is a must.

With this in mind, the development of the statistical group, and the education of the work force in statistics, can proceed in a fashion which reflects the relative need to understand statistics in depth. In Japan, everyone at every level understands statistics to a high degree. At FPL, everyone was taught statistics in courses which were quite exhaustive. The question which you will have to answer, depending on the resources available to you, will be how much emphasis to put on this difficult subject in return for the gain to be expected from doing it. At the moment, I believe that this may be more expeditiously done by focusing on process design, but this view may also change with time.

At this juncture, the TQM program can be announced to the work force inasmuch as there will be continuing activity at the top and middle levels. Training of the line personnel can begin under the QIDW group in conjunction with the quality council and outside consultants. Again, the work force gets the same training structure as anyone else with more focus on the practical aspects of process improvement. Following this initial training, the QIDW group, which has also been playing catchball with the quality council or translating the company goals of management by policy into departmental goals, will begin to work with the departments on identifying processes which are wholly owned by the departments and which need to be prioritized and stabilized. This is again done using the principal of catchball, this time played between the departments and the QIDW group. In the end, the departmental goals are both clearly defined and prioritized.

The next step is to work on interdepartmental alignment. This process addresses one of the major potential benefits from TQM at the department level—cross-functional goals. The processes which have shared ownership, or which cross over between departments, are now identified and prioritized in much the same way between the QIDW group and the departmental directors and managers. This ultimately results in a set of goals which reflect both intra- and interdepartmental needs. These are reprioritized under customer need categories such as quality, cost, and scheduling. These customer-derived needs, reflected at the departmental level, should be the center of the initial activity of TQM, and it goes without saying that the customer may be internal as well as external in this case.

Under the coordination of the QIDW group, the group activities can also begin. These can be both the quality circle activities as well as the task team projects directed by the priorities just established. In addition, since Imai says to think about the quality circles as a "group suggestion system," the suggestion structure needs to be in place and functioning to provide prompt response to any incoming thoughts from the line level or elsewhere.

EXECUTIVE PROCESS REVIEW

As the process of TQM begins to deploy throughout all levels and departments, there will be pockets of resistance. These may not necessarily be people who won't buy in, although this is possible, but people who remain allied to the tried-and-true methods which have brought them to where they are now. TQM is an unknown to them, and they see security in what they know and are comfortable with. To help stimulate change by rewarding good TQM group performance, the executive review is key to assuring that TQM is in place in all areas of the business.

At least once a year, but better semiannually, each department should be reviewed by the company president and his or her staff. Each department should either formally present, or be prepared to undergo informal review, of its progress under TQM to the present time. This process should be a two-way review in which the presidential staff not only reviews progress, but also asks what may be standing in the way to still greater improvement within the department.

Two things are accomplished by the review. First, senior management interest and support of the TQM program is exhibited by the review, which in many cases will be conducted in the departmental area if possible, and secondly, no one wants to go through such a review without positive results to show for the prior six months' of efforts in this area. Without the executive review, the deployment of TQM into all areas will be incomplete.

THE NEW ECONOMICS

TQM deployment maximizes the beneficial interaction of all the departments, divisions, levels, and groups, as well as suppliers and outside customers. The TQM process must center around the principle discussed under the Taguchi loss function—all area activities must be maximized. Project priorities must also keep this principle in mind. The smooth integration of all department processes and functions is the aim of TQM. One must be very careful not to maximize one domain at the expense of another. The harmonious interaction of all areas and functions is the goal.

Recently Dr. W. Edwards Deming was nominated for the Nobel Prize in Economics. Joseph Juran commented on this by saying that just as the Nobel Prize had outgrown Alfred Nobel, so had the Deming Prize outgrown its founder. Deming's new book called *The New Economics for Industry, Education, Government* builds on the concept just discussed and is portrayed in Figure 7.9. Deming believes that as businesses move into a total global economy, in which countries interact in a worldwide marketplace, cooperation rather than competition should be the aim. In this way, maximizing stockholder equity is not the key goal as it is now. Maximizing stockholder equity can be done by techniques such as laying off large numbers of people to dress up the company for sale as a lean-running organization, when, in fact, it is understaffed and won't be competitive for long in that condition. There are other ways, many of which are either customer neutral (certain productivity approaches), or employee indifferent, but generally both. These frequently work over a short time span, and if the investors are in and out before things pale, their goals have been met.

Instead, Deming advocates "maximizing the system of interdependent stakeholders" in the corporation. In this fashion, rather than win-lose, everyone with a stake in the company, from suppliers through customers,

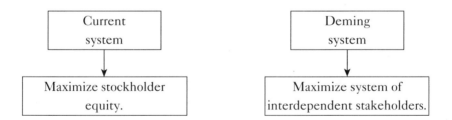

Figure 7.9: The new economics. Under traditional management systems, there is a vertical patronage from the employees up through supervision through to senior management. Eyes focused above, the president patronizes the CEO who patronizes the board members who patronize the stockholders. This sort of company loses sight of both the customer and the employee. Under the new paradigm, Deming depicts a business as being composed of an interdependent system of stakeholders. These include everyone from the suppliers through the workers, managers, executives, customers, consumers, and stockholders. Everyone is important and interdependent. The business runs best when all roles are maximized. If anyone is suboptimized, then the whole system suffers.

employers, and employees, are integrated in such a way that everyone wins. If any part of the integrated system is suboptimized, then the system suffers. This is akin to great music, and the perceptive comment made by Salieri in the movie *Amadeus* comes to mind. "Change one note, and there would be diminishment."

With strong, learned senior management you will be able to participate in a rewarding TQM effort. A member of the planning team which established the Federal Quality Institute put it this way, "TQM is the way we are going to conduct our business. It is not optional. All supervisors and managers will serve on and direct quality improvement teams. Improving the way we work is as important as doing our work well. The train is leaving the station. Get on board or get left on the platform."[3]

NOTES

1. Kersi F. Munshi, interview with author, August 1992. Also see Kersi F. Munshi, "The Importance of a Clear Corporate Vision in Policy Deployment," paper presented at the 1991 Juran Conference in Atlanta, Georgia, October 28–30, 1991. Munshi attributes the following mission statement to the Newport News shipyard in the seventeenth century, "We shall build good ships here—at a profit if we can, at a loss if we must—but always good ships."

2. Graham R. Wood and Kersi F. Munshi, "Hoshin Kanri: A Systematic Approach to Breakthrough Improvement," *Total Quality Management* 2, no. 3 (1991), 1–14.

3. Bob Carey, director of the Veterans' Affairs Regional Office and Insurance Center in John Scott McAllister, et al., *Federal TQM Handbook* (Washington, D.C.: Federal Quality Institute, 1991), 16. For more information, contact the Federal Quality Institute, PO Box 99, Washington D.C. 20044-0099; 202-376-3747.

Suggested Reading
Peter R. Scholtes, *The Team Handbook* (Madison, Wisc.: Joiner Associates, 1988). For more information, contact Joiner Associates, Inc., P.O. Box 5445, Madison, Wisconsin 53707; 608-238-8135 and 800-669-8326.

8

The Clinical
Laboratory from a
Regulatory Perspective

EXTERNAL CUSTOMERS

The clinical laboratory is a highly regulated industry. There are certain regulatory imperatives which are common to all businesses. These include state and local laws which may require either a certificate of occupancy, an occupational license, or both. These local laws may also reflect federal mandate at the local level. This is the situation where local regulations are in place to assure that the State meets federal requirements. An example is in the area of environmental control, where there may be local departments of environmental regulation which may promulgate directives sometimes more restrictive than federal ones, in order to protect a particularly sensitive environment. Figure 8.1 shows the bureaucratic relationship of the departments under Health and Human Services (HHS), which actively regulate the lab industry. Table 8.1 explores their regulatory mandate a little more closely.

In addition there are regulations which are not generally shared, but are focused specifically on the lab. These can include state licensing of lab

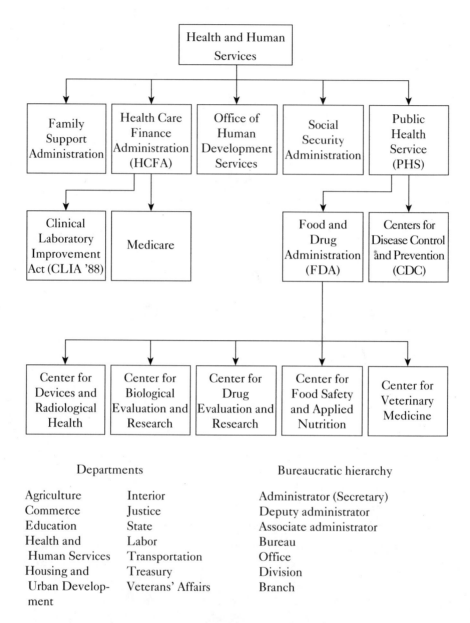

Departments		Bureaucratic hierarchy
Agriculture	Interior	Administrator (Secretary)
Commerce	Justice	Deputy administrator
Education	State	Associate administrator
Health and	Labor	Bureau
Human Services	Transportation	Office
Housing and	Treasury	Division
Urban Develop-	Veterans' Affairs	Branch
ment		

Figure 8.1: The Department of Health and Human Services.

personnel and lab operations, which may be more or less restrictive than federal licensing standards. In general, regulations can be divided into federal, state, and local, and the regulatory focus can center on the facility, the personnel, and the operations. In this section, the recent issues brought about by the CLIA '88, as administered by the HCFA, and the role of the U.S. FDA in the

Table 8.1: Federal agencies and their role in the laboratory.

Occupational Safety and Health Organization (OSHA): Relevant regulations include hazard communication, blood-borne pathogens, chemical hazard procedure, and general safe workplace.

Environmental Protection Agency (EPA): Regulations address the environment and the lab relationship to it via air and water (sewer).

Health Care Finance Administration (HCFA): HCFA is responsible for administering the Medicare program, as well as CLIA '88 which regulates all labs.

Food and Drug Administration (FDA): The FDA monitors the blood supply through its regulation of blood banks and plasma collection agencies and also plays the key role in clearing manufactured lab products for use in interstate commerce.

Centers for Disease Control and Prevention (CDC): In conjunction with HCFA and FDA, CDC is responsible for establishing the complexity of lab tests referenced in CLIA '88.

Bureau of Alcohol, Tobacco, and Firearms (ATF): Under the Department of the Treasury, any lab use of undenatured or specially denatured alcohol is registered with this bureau.

Nuclear Regulatory Commission (NRC): Certain large labs will require licensing under this agency for use of radioactive materials and will also require a radiation safety officer (RSO).

Drug Enforcement Agency (DEA): The use of certain restricted drugs in toxicology testing requires licensure with this agency.

United States Department of Agriculture (USDA): Any animal use such as hamsters, guinea pigs, rats, mice, cats, rabbits, and, of course, larger animals, requires licensure by this agency.

Department of Labor (DOL): The DOL regulates individuals working in the laboratory with regard to several statutes relating to wages, safety, age, and hours.

clinical lab will be explored. No in-depth analysis of either of these is intended; rather a view of the evolving issues through the new perspective of TQM is examined.

The perspective of TQM sheds some new light on some old issues, and may allow laboratorians to seek new solutions to some old problems.

Remember that the clinical lab can be viewed as a three-part system in which the input is instruments, reagents, and patient samples, and the output is reports to physicians, while the agency of transformation of input to output is the lab itself. It follows then that the regulations affecting the supply side of this system would have an impact on the entire system. Thus, the regulations affecting the suppliers of lab equipment are quite important since excessive or inappropriate regulation adds cost which is passed along to the lab, which is further passed on to those who pay for lab services. This can be patients, insurance companies, or in the case of Medicare and Medicaid, all taxpayers.

In 1987, the FDA circulated a tentative regulation indicating a major shift in emphasis from the routine techniques it used to assure the safety and effectiveness of diagnostic procedures, kits, and components. Manufacturers which supply clinical laboratories have, since 1976, been under FDA regulations, a portion of which are referred to as the current Good Manufacturing Practices or cGMPs. These sections of the Code of Federal Regulations (CFR) define minimal standards with which manufacturers must comply in order to continue doing business with the labs. These standards then directly impact on the development, delivery, timeliness, and quality of products in routine use in clinical laboratories in the United States.

One shortcoming of many current regulatory change systems is lack of prior data to compare with what is generated by the new regulations. To give the writers of CLIA '88 credit, data gathering was required by the regulations. The studies that were required were designed to assess such things as the relationship between lab performance and performance on proficiency testing, and amount and type of personnel training and education as this related to lab performance. The experimental design was relegated to a group in North Carolina which presented a design, and since that time not much has been heard. So, what metrics were chosen and how they will affect future regulation are still being determined. The principle, however, is a good one; management by data, tracking change and process improvement through a choice of the proper metrics, and the judicious use of these appraisals.

The FDA needs a mission statement from which the FDA could derive an operational system which protects the consumer from products which are not safe and effective, but does it in such a way that U.S. companies can continue to be competitive in the world market. Currently, the incentive is for large manufacturers to operate outside of the United States to avoid regulatory burden.

That this attitude is shared by others in high places was recently brought to the public's attention by then-President George Bush. He announced on January 20, 1992 that in an attempt to jump start a floundering U.S. economy, he was placing a moratorium on all new regulations for an undetermined time until the economy could dig its way out from under the already oppressive burden of too many regulations and not enough productivity. President Bush also established a council on productivity run by Vice-President Quayle, which was essentially an antiregulatory think tank. President Clinton abolished this operation saying "The back door is closed." Truly it should be, but the front door should be more widely open, and currently that isn't the case. What I mean by this is that creating more bureaucracy to derail existing bureaucracy isn't the answer. The answer is to structure, focus, and correctly manage the existing organizations to better serve the public.

The FDA requires that manufacturers show that their products are safe and effective through arduous premarket approval processes. There is, unfortunately, no requirement that the FDA be similarly controlled when launching new policy. Currently, there is never any real way to tell if the system change the FDA launches ever results in any improvement in manufacturer delivery because no data are taken before or after the FDA implements the change. This is a classic example of repeating the PD part of the PDCA cycle with no check component; that is, no evaluation of whether the process change is resulting in improvement or not. Many people who have worked under the GMPs since they were implemented believe that they have had no positive effect on the quality of reagents and test kits used in the laboratory, but result in the most recent technologies being made available everywhere else in the world except in the United States. With the lack of supporting data to the contrary, there is no way to dispute this. It has resulted in the widely known saying, "Who is watching the watchers, while the watchers are out watching?"

In the spirit of TQM, the FDA elected to shift emphasis from end-process and in-process control checks to process validation. Since 21 CFR 820 don't specifically mention this, FDA claimed that it was "implicit" in the regulations and that it was going to change the GMPs anyway to make it more explicit. As this book goes to press the process is still ongoing, and it has been stated that the new cGMPs will more closely reflect a set of international standards called ISO 9000 criteria, which will be closely examined later in this chapter.

The FDA emphasis on process validation is in keeping with TQM thinking from two viewpoints. The first is that the focus is on the process rather than inspection, and the second is that, because validation implies scheduled revalidation, this can be tied to process improvement. Revalidation then should result in something other than another increase in the already oppressive regulatory burden under which diagnostic manufacturers and clinical labs operate.

CLIA '88 has a good section calling for a quality assurance program. This new regulatory aspect also incorporates a system focus rather than the older QC function. Prior regulatory concentration was on quality control and the use of proficiency testing to verify acceptable lab operation. The new quality assurance (QA) section is broader. Laboratorians had been taught earlier that analytical error was divided into random and systematic, and that systematic error was further divided into constant and proportional error. This focus, although it brought some good things, was far too tight in terms of the overall quality of the lab output. The new CLIA '88 QA section clearly recognizes that the lab has "preanalytic, analytic, and postanalytic" components, and that all three contribute to a good lab operation and should be reviewed on a scheduled basis. To help see this process in more detail, I have included two procedures in the appendices. The first is a protocol for structuring general procedures (Appendix A), and the second is a protocol addressing the QA section of CLIA '88 (Appendix B).

Unfortunately CLIA '88 seems to be going into the history books as one of the classic pieces of bad legislation of the 20th century. Certainly the lab-owner physicians hate it, and President Clinton may yet steer them clear of the legislation as he garners physician support for his health care reform package. It is interesting that the plan's architect, Dr. Gail Wilenski, went over to the White House to run President Bush's health care reform. The ex-president's health care reform consisted of tax credits which the public would take to the existing market to pursue more of what the system currently offers.

The fact that health care was a major campaign issue stemmed from nearly universal agreement that this is a system badly in need of improvement. A badly designed and managed system will not improve with an influx of additional funding. In the case of the current health care system, more money chasing the same services will result in another inflationary turn with no improvement in the quality of the delivery.

Since the FDA, CLIA '88, and Medicare fall under HHS, the secretary of HHS has a unique opportunity to coordinate these regulatory bodies, and convert their efforts into a cooperative process. Here, the regulators would operate in harmony with, rather than in opposition to, the health care business community.

To keep this country from slipping into a third-world status takes everyone's efforts. Everyone must understand TQM and tell the representatives in

Congress that these methods must be used not just in the business community but also in government. President Bush issued an executive order mandating that TQM be integrated with the federal bureaucracy, and this occasioned the publication of a series of TQM booklets available from the Federal Quality Institute (see chapter 7 notes). This was supported by President Clinton who assigned the task to Vice-President Gore. Clinton also said that he saw the federal government in a partnership with U.S. industry to regain world leadership. This would be good. Hope springs eternal.

PROCESS VALIDATION

Process validation was part of the CLIA '67 regulations. Process validation was again required in the combined regulations (42 CFR 493.1215, *Federal Register* March 14, 1990). To bring the final CLIA '88 regs more into keeping with the GMPs, the term *validation* was replaced by "verify and establish performance characteristics," and the standards put forth became part of section 1213. Also, for the first time, FDA requirements are explicitly expressed in CLIA '88, inasmuch as labs are expected, in certain cases, to default to the manufacturer's package insert protocol. This protocol is generally a compromise between what the diagnostic manufacturer has initially proposed and what the FDA reviewers feel is in keeping with FDA priorities. The outcome is that the clinical labs ultimately are marching to the tune of the FDA which, prior to CLIA '88, had no regulatory aegis over the labs. This is risky because it does not give lab professionals the flexibility to correct oversights or to add ancillary control procedures which may be appropriate to their clinical setting. No agreement reached between a manufacturer and the FDA on a package insert can ever anticipate all of the circumstances under which a diagnostic is used in the lab. It is unfortunate that CLIA '88 fosters this belief.

The theory behind process validation rests in Deming's third point, "cease dependence on final inspection." In the Japanese operation, control charts are not used to the extent process control is. Consider a diagnostic product which is filled into vials for final distribution as a liquid product. Despite the addition of antibiotics and preservatives, it is important that the product be filled as microbe-free as possible. This is conventionally verified by sampling the filled product and testing it for bacterial, mycotic, and sometimes viral growth. The microbial contaminants are removed by a filtration scheme which generally uses different grades of filters starting with a coarse prefilter and ending with a tight final filter frequently in the range of 0.2 μm absolute or tighter.

The problem with relying on the final vial check for microbial content is that the lot is released based on a sampling plan which selects a statistically reasonable sample of the vials and subjects them to sterility testing. This gives a certain probability that the lot is fine. If the filling process has special-cause variability, however, then samples, generally selected from the beginning, middle, and end of the filling process, may not truly reflect the overall fill, because the fill may not be homogeneous. The FDA feels then, that if the filling process is validated, that is, all the process components are optimized and documented as being in control, then the final microbial check will be relegated to a gross check of whether or not a filter was blown during fill. This is in place of any assessment of the quality of the fill.

Figure 8.2 shows a flowchart of the validation process. The process can be broken down into eight major steps beginning with the process specifications, that is, what the process is supposed to be delivering. To paraphrase the FDA: Process validation is establishing documented evidence which provides a high degree of assurance that a specified process will consistently meet its predetermined specifications and quality characteristics.

Regarding the second step of the validation process, the test protocol, the FDA says,[1] "It is important that the manufacturer prepare a written validation protocol which specifies the procedures and tests to be conducted and the data to be collected." In the combined CLIA '88–Medicare regs, it says, "A method used by a laboratory must be validated before it is used and documentation of the validation must be available. . . . The laboratory must have documentation of the level of precision, accuracy, sensitivity, and specificity that the laboratory claims for each method in use." The latter language appeared in the final CLIA '88 regs, and it is for any new lab procedure or for any modification of an existing procedure.

The FDA goes on to specify key elements it believes to be important in the protocol. These include the following:

1. Use a sufficient number of replicate process runs to demonstrate reproducibility.
2. Utilize test conditions that encompass upper and lower processing limits and circumstances. (CLIA '88 reflects over the linear range of assay.)
3. Apply "worst case" conditions or "most appropriate challenge" conditions. For instance, in validating an autoclave, choose the longest cycle time and heaviest load.

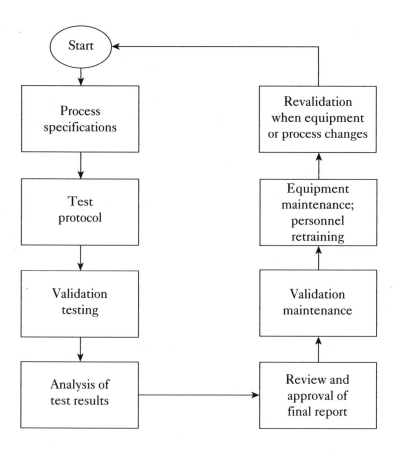

Figure 8.2: Process validation flowchart.

4. Include evidence of the suitability of materials (reagents, kits) and the performance reliability of equipment and systems.

When actually doing the validation testing per protocol, the FDA recommends monitoring the key process variables which will have been identified in the protocol, and that "analysis of the data collected from monitoring will establish the variability of process parameters for individual runs and will establish whether or not the equipment and process controls are adequate to assure that . . . specifications are met."[2]

Clearly two lessons from TQM must be applied to this analysis. One is the 6-M process components given in the Ishikawa diagram, and the other is to design the protocol with a statistical completeness in mind so that the data analysis rests on firm statistical ground. Without these two elements in mind, process components may be overlooked and the data will not validate the process performance to an acceptable degree if statistical reduction is not contemplated appropriately in the validation process design. This falls under the area of one of the advanced QC tools, design of experiments.

Following data collection, the study should be reviewed and approved. The sign-off approval for the process validation should include the supervisory representatives from the group responsible for the protocol design, those who conducted the testing, and the process owners.

At this time it is appropriate to write a revalidation protocol. The schedule for the revalidation studies may be derived from observations made during the validation testing. Not only time, but extent of revalidation testing, need to be determined. This is as important from the TQM perspective as the original validation and will assure ongoing process maintenance and improvement. Revalidation should be done when the equipment or process is changed sufficiently to no longer reflect the data collection of the initial validation process.

The procedure just described is what the FDA calls a "prospective validation." It assumes a new process (or for manufacturers, a product made from component processes). As the FDA emphasis refocuses on process validation, and HCFA, through CLIA '88, begins to require it also, many ongoing processes will need validation. FDA calls this a "retrospective validation." In this case, following protocol development, data may be collected from past performance, and, assuming that past performance as delivering what was needed, the steps of statistical reduction, review approval, documentation, and revalidation are applicable.

A third type of validation is "concurrent validation." FDA originally saw this as applicable to a one-time, custom-designed, ad hoc product or process, in which the in-process and end-process checks of the ongoing process would be given much more emphasis than prospective or retrospective issues. In a broader sense though, the FDA sees this as an ongoing process adjunctive to the retrospective audit inasmuch "As additional data is gathered on production lots, such data can be used to build confidence in the adequacy of the process. Conversely, such data may indicate a declining confidence in the process and a commensurate need for corrective changes." Sections 1211(16)(g) and 1221 of CLIA require that these records be kept for as long as the process is being used in the lab, or for two years, whichever is longer, unless the records relate to immunohematology in which case the more extensive FDA requirements of 21 CFR 606.160 apply.

ISO 9000

ISO 9000 is the generic name for a set of standards and guidance documents adopted in 1987 by the International Organization for Standardization. Over 50 countries have now adopted these standards, and the U.S. member organization is the American National Standards Institute (ANSI). The relevance to the lab is that the FDA is adopting these standards into the GMPs and these are to be issued shortly. In addition, many diagnostic manufacturing companies which see ISO 9000 registration as a requirement for marketing overseas are integrating these standards into their own TQM programs, or using the ISO standards as a starting point for their quality efforts.

The most comprehensive standard document is ISO 9001, and the table of contents of that document is reprinted in Table 8.2. The standard outlines 20 separate areas to be addressed in the quality system. A companion guidance document, ISO 9004, explains these standards in more detail, and the contents of that document is reproduced in Table 8.3. For a modest charge, a full set of these documents can be obtained from ASQC and is known as the Q90 series.

These guidelines have been adopted largely by the European Community (EC), which is badly in need of standardization. In Europe, the electric power voltage and frequency change from country to country as well as the currency, language, and customs. As a result, Europe, as a unit, is in the SDCA cycle of TQM deployment. Recall that a system must be standardized before process improvement can begin. Although Europe badly needs this standardization, it is totally superfluous in the Japanese community and little needed in the United States as well.

The EC, however, may use the ISO standards as a nontariff trade barrier, and this will mandate certification of those companies wanting to do business there. As an example, IBM recently closed a sale of $300 million worth of computers to Denmark. Denmark refused delivery stating that IBM wasn't ISO 9001 certified. IBM replied by saying that the computers had been built in Scotland at an ISO 9001 certified division, so pay up. Denmark retorted that the computers had been designed in Houston which wasn't certified, so forget it. Since the design category is included in the ISO 9001 standard, IBM had to get the Houston plant certified. When that was done, Denmark took the computers. Fear of similar circumstances in other industries is creating considerable interest here.

The question sometimes arises as to the difference between the ISO standards and the Baldrige criteria. The latter are considerably more

Table 8.2: ISO 9001 quality system requirements.

4.1 Management responsibility
      4.1.1. Quality policy
      4.1.2. Organization
            4.1.2.1. Responsibility and authority
            4.1.2.2. Verification resources and personnel
            4.1.2.3. Management representative
      4.1.3. Management review
4.2. Quality system
4.3. Contract review
4.4. Design control
      4.4.1. General
      4.4.2. Design and development planning
            4.4.2.1. Activity assignment
            4.4.2.2. Organizational and technical interfaces
      4.4.3. Design input
      4.4.4. Design output
      4.4.5. Design verification
      4.4.6. Design changes
4.5. Document control
      4.5.1. Document approval and issue
      4.5.2. Document changes/modifications
4.6. Purchasing
      4.6.1. General
      4.6.2. Assessment of subcontractors
      4.6.3. Purchasing data
      4.6.4. Verification of purchased product
4.7. Purchaser supplied product
4.8. Product identification and traceability
4.9. Process control
      4.9.1. General
      4.9.2. Special processes
4.10. Inspection and testing
      4.10.1. Receiving inspection and testing
            4.10.1.1. Routine use quarantine
            4.10.1.2. Emergency use conditions
      4.10.2. In-process inspection and testing
      4.10.3. Final inspection and testing
      4.10.4. Inspection and test records
4.11. Inspection, measuring, and test equipment
4.12. Inspection and test status
4.13. Control of nonconforming product
      4.13.1. Nonconformity review and disposition
4.14. Corrective action

continued

Table 8.2: *continued*

4.15. Handling, storage, packaging, and delivery
        4.15.1. General
        4.15.2. Handling
        4.15.3. Storage
        4.15.4. Packaging
        4.15.5. Delivery
4.16. Quality records
4.17. Internal quality audits
4.18. Training
4.19. Servicing
4.20. Statistical techniques

comprehensive and incorporate the customer focus as well as a companywide quality system which requires continuous improvement. The Baldrige is also results oriented which the ISO standards do not address. As a Baldrige examiner I reviewed two companies which were ISO certified. One was light years away from meeting the Baldrige criteria, and the other was excellent. I wouldn't be at all surprised to see the second company win the Baldrige in the near future. So although there are common elements in the two standards, they are not mutually inclusive. Being ISO 9000 certified doesn't preclude a total quality management system, but it doesn't assure that there will be one.

INTEGRATING SERVICES IN THE LAB INDUSTRY

When W. Edwards Deming addressed the country via satellite downlink from George Washington University in the fall of 1991, he spoke for several hours on his management thoughts and observed that the Japanese have done rather well after adopting them. One comment he made had particular relevance to recent events affecting the clinical laboratory. Deming said, "We have been misled by economists who say that competition is good. Competition is bad. What we need is more cooperation. We shouldn't be seeking a greater percentage of market share. We should be seeking new markets."

Deming then went on to use examples such as "every hospital having to have all of the latest diagnostic equipment." A corollary to that statement is that there is no shortage of hospital administrators who feel strongly that a shortage of equipment will lead to a shortage of physicians and their patients. Deming, however, has always said that as far as existing markets

Table 8.3: ISO 9004 quality management and quality system guidelines.

4.0. Management responsibility
      4.1. General
      4.2. Quality policy
      4.3. Quality objectives
      4.4. Quality system
5.0. Quality system principles
      5.1. Quality loop
      5.2. Structure of the quality system
            5.2.1. General
            5.2.2. Quality responsibility and authority
            5.2.3. Organizational structure
            5.2.4. Resources and personnel
            5.2.5. Operational procedures
      5.3. Documentation of the system
            5.3.1. Quality policies and procedures
            5.3.2. Quality manual
            5.3.3. Quality plans
            5.3.4. Quality records
      5.4. Auditing the quality system
            5.4.1. General
            5.4.2. Audit plan
            5.4.3. Carrying out the audit
            5.4.4. Reporting and follow-up of audit findings
      5.5. Review and evaluation of the quality management system
6.0 Economics—quality-related cost considerations
      6.1. General
      6.2. Selecting appropriate elements
      6.3. Types of quality-related costs
            6.3.1. General
            6.3.2. Operating quality costs
            6.3.3. External assurance quality costs
      6.4. Management visibility
7.0 Quality in marketing
      7.1. Marketing requirements
      7.2. Product brief
      7.3. Customer feedback information
8.0 Quality in specification and design
      8.1. Contribution of specification and design to quality
      8.2. Design planning and objectives (defining the project)
      8.3. Product testing and measurement
      8.4. Design qualification and validation

continued

Table 8.3: *continued*

8.5. Design review
    8.5.1. General
    8.5.2. Elements of design reviews
        8.5.2.a. Customer needs and satisfaction
        8.5.2.b. Product specification and service requirements
        8.5.2.c. Process specifications and service requirements
    8.5.3. Design verification
8.6. Design baseline and production release
8.7. Market readiness review
8.8. Design change control (configuration management)
9.0. Quality in Procurement
    9.1. General
    9.2. Requirements for specifications, drawings, and purchase orders
    9.3. Selection of qualified suppliers
    9.4. Agreement on quality assurance
    9.5. Agreement on verification methods
    9.6. Provision for settlement of quality disputes
    9.7. Receiving inspection planning and controls
    9.8. Receiving quality records
10.0. Quality in production
    10.1. Planning for controlled production
    10.2. Process capability
    10.3. Supplies, utilities, and environments
11.0. Control of production
    11.1. General
    11.2. Materials and traceability
    11.3. Equipment control and maintenance
    11.4. Special processes
    11.5. Documentation
    11.6. Process change control
    11.7. Control of verification status
    11.8. Control of nonconforming materials
12.0. Product verification
    12.1. Incoming materials and parts
    12.2. In-process inspection
    12.3. Completed product verification
13.0. Control of measuring and test equipment
    13.1. Measurement control

continued

Table 8.3: *continued*

13.2. Elements of control
13.3. Supplier measurement controls
13.4. Corrective action
13.5. Outside testing
14.0. Conformity
  14.1. General
  14.2. Identification
  14.3. Segregation
  14.4. Review
  14.5. Disposition
  14.6. Documentation
  14.7. Prevention of recurrence
15.0. Corrective action
  15.1. General
  15.2. Assignment of responsibility
  15.3. Evaluation of importance
  15.4. Investigation of possible causes
  15.5. Analysis of problem
  15.6. Preventive action
  15.7. Process controls
  15.8. Disposition of nonconforming items
  15.9. Permanent changes
16.0. Handling and post-production functions
  16.1. Handling, storage, identification, packaging, installation, and delivery
  16.2. After-sales servicing
  16.3. Marketing reporting and product supervision
17.0. Quality documentation and records
18.0. Personnel
  18.1. Training
    18.1.1. General
    18.1.2. Executive and management personnel
    18.1.3. Technical personnel
    18.1.4. Production supervisors and workers
  18.2. Qualification
  18.3. Motivation.
    18.3.1. General
    18.3.2. Application
    18.3.3. Quality awareness
    18.3.4. Measuring quality
19.0 Product safety and liability
20.0 Use of statistical methods
  20.1. Applications
  20.2. Statistical techniques

go, cooperation is, in the long range, more effective than competition, and that resources would be better used opening up new areas rather than in the endless struggle for territoriality.

Another example that comes to mind is the recently enacted "shell laboratory" provision. This is a federal enforcement activity directed at labs doing Medicare work. It is a program which is interesting from a TQM perspective.

A clinical laboratory cannot order a clinical lab test. Only physicians can do that. In effect then, Medicare can't be billed more than once for a test at prevailing rates. It doesn't matter who bills for the test—the doctor, the shell lab, or the performing lab—Medicare only gets billed once at a figure it controls.

The reason direct billing by the laboratory came into being was to thwart the only potential abuse, that of overutilization by the physician who was able to bill Medicare and order tests. Recent studies indicate that this abuse happened often enough to be a problem. There is no wish to curtail the ordering of tests at any frequency by the physician. But if tests are being ordered too frequently for whatever reason, then the taxpayers shouldn't have to underwrite them. Consequently, direct billing became a reality. Under this system, only the lab could bill Medicare, and since the lab couldn't order, the potential for overutilization went away. There were, however, some loopholes. The regulation didn't specify that the billing lab had to be the one doing the work, and it didn't limit ownership of the labs in any way.

In reaction to direct billing, physicians set up their own office labs (POLs), and this new market was supported enthusiastically by instrument and reagent manufacturers with a wave of POL lab equipment and supplies. Physician-owned shell labs also came into being so that the shell lab could continue to bill Medicare, while passing on the work to reference labs who charged much less. The profit could be built into the difference between what was billed Medicare and what the lab charged. Since the Medicare allowable was capped, increasing profits meant using predatory pricing methods on the reference labs.

Intended to neutralize these strategies were three pieces of legislation, CLIA '88, the Stark Ethics in Self-Referral legislation, and the shell lab provisions. None of these legislative pieces limited what testing physicians could order or how often. The question was always one of reimbursement, and if the patients or their insurance companies would pay, no problem. If Medicare was billed, however, the shell lab provision said that the lab had to be doing 70 percent of relevant testing, ethics in self-referral said the lab had to be for the physician's own patients only, and CLIA said that the lab had to be licensed and had to do proficiency testing.

Feeling that this was still too restrictive, physicians and diagnostic manufacturers lobbied for surcease. The timing was good inasmuch as President Clinton and his wife Hillary Rodham Clinton were looking for support of their health care reform package from the medical constituency, and trading off concessions on POL restrictions has been offered to the medical community as inducement. This is continuing as of this writing. In the spirit of TQM, it is hoped that physicians can order tests they feel are medically appropriate, and do them in any facility that offers the public quality work.

Prior abuse, however, resulted in the shell lab provisions and the ethics in self-referral legislation. As the Chinese say, "When things go wrong, first look in the mirror."

An earlier chapter emphasized the 80/20 relationship of Pareto analysis, in which 80 percent of system variation may be caused by 20 percent of the possible causes, which leads to prioritization in systems analysis and remediation. Dr. Vincent K. Omachonu, in his book *Total Quality and Productivity Management in Health Care Organizations*, points out that a similar 80/20 rule applies specifically to health care. Eighty percent of health care expenditures are directly attributable to physician directives. Omachonu says " Eighty percent of medical care expenditures are for services prescribed by physicians despite the fact that physician's fees represent only about 20 percent of health care costs. Physicians drive almost every aspect of the demand for health care."

The United States currently spends 12 percent of its gross national product (GNP) on health care. At the present rate of increase in health care spending, *all* of the GNP will go into health care in about 50 years. Americans seem to want a high quality system to assure this type of service. Crucial to this service are the attending physicians. To exploit the system at the expense of the public, however, won't do. For the system to work, the physician must participate in a professional and responsible manner. To do otherwise is to warrant the cynicism of the public and invite increased regulatory pressure directed at any business venture with potential for abusing the public trust.

It may be, however, that HCFA, in fishing around for an effective method to curtail these abuses, cast its net too wide. The result is that the shell lab proviso curtails legitimate integration of lab testing efforts in keeping with Deming's counsel about the need for cooperation within an industry.

The hospital or community lab may not need all of the latest testing equipment and staffing to meet the community's highly specialized testing needs. So it may fill these needs based on more common tests, referring the more highly specialized or more difficult analyses to the reference laboratory. In this fashion, the community is served by prompt dispatch of more commonly ordered testing, and the specialty lab fills a role by performing within areas of its own expertise. The effect on Medicare is transparent, since it is billed once and no incentive exists for overutilization.

The shell lab stipulations may cause this effective and sensible integration to fail resulting in duplication of equipment and services and unfairly prohibiting the community lab from billing for appropriate charges. The solution is to enforce the ethics in self-referral provisions, and the shell lab provision becomes redundant and unneccessary.

USING THE BALDRIGE CRITERIA
TO STRUCTURE A TQM PROGRAM

At the 25th anniversary meeting of the National Committee for Clinical Laboratory Standards (NCCLS) held March 25, 1993, in Baltimore, a representative of the Joint Commission on the Accreditation of Healthcare Organizations (JCAHO) announced that it would be using the Malcolm Baldrige National Quality Award (MBNQA) guidelines for certification. The representative said that compliance with these guidelines would be required by 1996. This announcement was greeted with acclaim in many quality management quarters, because now the hospitals would have a set of guidelines which were clear and traceable directly to a great body of supporting literature, which also showed ways to increase productivity and reduce costs.

JCAHO subsequently backed away from this position citing the Baldrige focus on for-profit activities among other concerns. Note that the Baldrige administrators continue to consider widening the categories to include nonprofit activities, their rationale being that a quality effort should be judged as such irrespective of the business segment from which it derives. Further, the state of Florida has the Sterling Award, an award modeled after the Baldrige award, which already includes nonprofit activities. In 1993 of the four Sterling awards that were given, one went to AT&T Universal Card Services, which has previously won the Baldrige award, and another went to the Pinellas County School District. The latter would not be able to apply for the Baldrige under 1994 guidelines, but this didn't stop the district from launching a first-rate TQM program based on Deming principles.

Dr. Don Berwick is the president of the Institute for Healthcare Improvement (IHI) in Boston. Dr. Berwick wrote a book with A. Blanton

Godfrey, CEO of the Juran Institute, called *Curing Healthcare*.[3] Associated with IHI is a group of 32 hospitals known as the Quality Management Network which is studying JCAHO/MBNQA integration. The executive director of that network is Francis Jackson, also an MBNQA examiner. As we go to print the study is ongoing but should yield some good information on the potential of the JCAHO/MBNQA interface.

Irrespective of what the final JCAHO position on this issue might be, the use of the MBNQA criteria to structure a quality management program within a hospital setting is certainly an appropriate approach. This cannot only accommodate current regulatory requirements, but it is also much more likely to generate a quality output than efforts which address regulatory requirements only. In this sense then, the following example of the lab role in a hospital setting using the Baldrige criteria is presented to illustrate how this might be done. In the telling, I share some of my own perspective and experience as a member of the Board of Examiners of the MBNQA.

INTRODUCTION TO THE BALDRIGE CRITERIA

The seven major categories of the Baldrige award are as follows:

1.0. Leadership
2.0. Information and analysis
3.0. Strategic quality planning
4.0. Human resource development and management
5.0. Management of process quality
6.0. Quality and operational results
7.0. Customer focus and satisfaction

Each of these categories is divided so that there are 28 major categories which are then further broken down into a total of 98 subsections overall. These categories, with their associated point total are shown in Table 8.4. The MBNQA was established in 1987, and the responsibility for administering the award was assigned to the Department of Commerce. The award is administered by an agency of the department, the National Institute of Standards and Technology (formerly the National Bureau of Standards). Assisting in the administration is the ASQC, which handles all of the communications during the scoring and evaluation process. This protects the confidentiality of the companies' submissions from public scrutiny under

Table 8.4: The MBNQA examination categories (1994).

Category	Points
1.0. Leadership	
1.1. Senior executive leadership	45
1.2. Management for quality	25
1.3. Public responsibility and corporate citizenship	25
2.0. Information and analysis	
2.1. Scope and management of performance data and information	15
2.2. Competitive comparisons and benchmarking	20
2.3. Analysis and uses of company level data	40
3.0. Strategic quality planning	
3.1. Strategic planning and company performance planning process	35
3.2. Quality and performance plans	25
4.0. Human resource development and management	
4.1. Human resource planning and management	20
4.2. Employee involvement	40
4.3. Employee education and training	40
4.4. Employee performance and recognition	25
4.5. Employee well-being and satisfaction	25
5.0. Management of process quality	
5.1. Design and introduction of quality products and services	40
5.2. Process management: product and service production and delivery processes	35
5.3. Process management: business processes and support services	30
5.4. Supplier quality	20
5.5. Quality assessment	15
6.0. Quality and operational results	
6.1. Product and service quality results	70
6.2. Company operational results	50
6.3. Business process and support service results	25
6.4. Supplier quality results	35
7.0. Customer focus and satisfaction	
7.1. Customer expectations: current and future	35
7.2. Customer relationship management	65
7.3. Commitment to customers	15
7.4. Customer satisfaction determination	30
7.5. Customer satisfaction results	85
7.6. Customer satisfaction comparison	70
Total	1000

the Freedom of Information Act. Confidentiality and image are the twin pillars of the MBNQA. Examiners are encouraged to talk in general about the process, but are proscribed from revealing any specific details of what companies they reviewed or any related details.

General Background

Figure 8.3 shows how the seven Baldrige categories are thought to be related in a business setting. Section 1.0, Leadership, is seen as the driver of the system, and the system itself is composed of the next four sections. The Baldrige is a results-oriented award since the Department of Commerce does not particularly want to hold up as an example to the rest of the business community a company which is responsive to all TQM criteria, but not performing well financially. Consequently, the last two sections of the MBNQA relate primarily to operation results and customer satisfaction. The following discourse uses examples from the hospital lab setting. Also, the quotation at the beginning of each section is taken directly from the introductory material in the Baldrige criteria booklet.

Leadership (1.0)

The leadership category examines senior executives' *personal* leadership and involvement in creating and sustaining a customer focus and clear and visible quality values. Also examined is how the quality values are integrated into the company's management system and reflected in the manner in which the company addresses its public responsibilities and corporate citizenship.

Section 1.0 is directed at senior executive leadership. The hospital lab may have little representation in this area, but the key to compliance with the MBNQA criteria is to think of the lab as a stand-alone microcosm which shares all the characteristics of a business. The three sections under this criterion are senior executive leadership, management for quality, and public responsibility and corporate citizenship. The lab must respond with its own mission and vision statements which are linked to those of the hospital. The formal TQM training of the lab leaders must be documented as is their role in disseminating this knowledge throughout the lab and throughout the community. All activities must be documented. For instance, if the lab directors state that they spend 35 percent of their time on TQM-related activities, the first thing an examiner would request during a site visit, would be the leaders' personal planner to review the type and frequency of these activities.

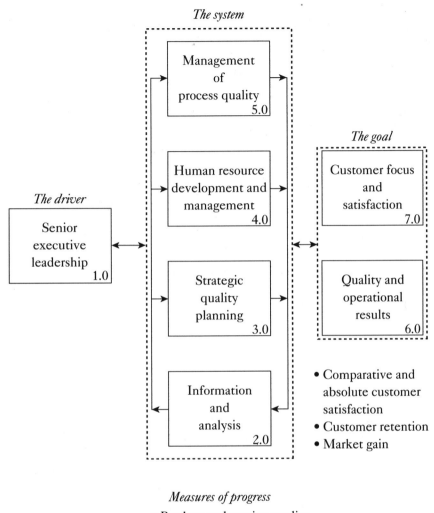

The system

Management
of
process quality
5.0

The goal

Customer focus
and
satisfaction
7.0

Human resource
development and
management
4.0

The driver

Senior
executive
leadership
1.0

Strategic
quality
planning
3.0

Quality and
operational
results
6.0

Information
and
analysis
2.0

• Comparative and
   absolute customer
   satisfaction
• Customer retention
• Market gain

Measures of progress
• Product and service quality
• Productivity improvement
• Waste reduction
• Supplier quality

Figure 8.3: Baldrige award criteria framework: dynamic relationships.

Right up front, the MBNQA asks for the means by which the senior level planning functions are integrated into the company's management system. What is sought here is a system akin to hoshin kanri (target and means control), known in this country as hoshin planning, management by policy, or policy management. Whatever the name, it is a formal structure for integrating and coordinating the company direction with management activities. Lack of this coordination will result in what some of the Baldrige examiners call the "popcorn effect," where one activity will jump up, call for prioritization, followed by another random surfacing, and so forth with no coherent effort aimed at prioritizing or coordinating these activities. This is what Lee Iacocca characterized as "management by swarm" when he first arrived at Ford. As he put it, a problem would be identified, and managers would swarm on it "like linebackers on a fumble." This is quite typical of command and control management systems where the intent is to impress management with one's enthusiasm rather than having any organized plan for the improvement of product and service delivery.

Information and Analysis (2.0)

The information and analysis category examines the scope, validity, analysis, management, and use of data and information to drive quality excellence and to improve operational and competitive performance. Also examined is the adequacy of the company's data, information, and analysis system to support improvement of the company's customer focus, products, services, and internal operations.

TQM is frequently referred to as management by data, as opposed to traditional management styles which rely more on intuition and prior experience. To reflect this, the lab's ability to collect information and data and to integrate it into process improvement will be key. Computer capability such as the local area network (LAN) and the lab information management system (LIMS) will be reviewed. The breadth and depth of the information, particularly customer-related information, and its use in planning are reviewed here. A great deal of information not readily obtainable will have to be collected. This is information which relates to lab process delivery, the customer perception of the output, and the financial ramifications of the overall process.

The concept of benchmarking appears for the first time in this section. Benchmarking is used to direct the degree of a process improvement activity. To remain competitive, a process improvement must be implemented which results in improvement better than the industry average, and hopefully equivalent to world-class performance. Neither of these benchmark indicators is routinely available, and so it would behoove the industry to undertake cooperative data-gathering efforts which would make this information accessible.

Strategic Quality Planning (3.0)

The strategic quality planning category examines the company's planning process and how all key quality requirements are integrated into overall business planning. Also examined are the company's short- and longer-term plans and how quality and operational performance requirements are deployed to all work units.

The two sections in this category first address the quality planning process and then the resultant plans themselves. In this section all inputs to the planning process must be considered including customer input, senior management input, supplier input, user (customer) input, and both individual and group employee input. The hospital mission and vision statements will have to be linked to the lab plans through the hoshin planning process which incorporates the strategic business plan (SBP) and quality function deployment. In this way, the vision of management and the voice of the customer are linked to the hospital capabilities, which include personnel, facilities, equipment, and financial resources. In assessing the efficacy of the planning process, the reviewer will look for the intelligent use of the planning tools and, most importantly, an integrated management structure which consolidates the planning efforts in a coordinated fashion.

The output of this planning, the plans themselves, should reflect short-term (one to two years) and long-term (more than three years) projections. This is the first use of the terms *key quality factors* and *key operational performance requirements*. The key quality factors are the services the lab must provide to excite and delight its customers, and the performance characteristics are the operational systems needed to support the service delivery. At a minimum, the plans should address the key cross-functional quality components of cost, scheduling, quality, and safety.

The first three cross-functional components were identified as being common elements which customers consider fundamental to a superior service or product. To address these items, the lab must concentrate on its productivity or its ability to deliver its services cost effectively. In addition, a quality service is not highly valued if it is not delivered when the customer wants it. This is called scheduling or delivery. The point is to shorten turnaround time and to make available the scheduling of send outs so that decisions can be made consistent with the delivery of lab results. Further, the quality of these lab services are determined by the user, and this includes the types of testing done and the locations at which the testing is made available.

Safety is not a key customer requirement. This is an issue which is transparent to the customer. It is a cross-functional concern and a regulatory requirement, however, and companies which have a strong program in this area are highly regarded.

Thinking in terms of the Deming wheel, the Baldrige criteria include human resources as a major component of the planning function in section 4.0. Section 5.0 addresses the do function and how these plans are implemented.

Human Resource Development and Management (4.0)

The human resource development and management category examines the key elements of how the work force is enabled to develop its full potential to pursue the company's quality and operational performance objectives. Also examined are the company's efforts to build and maintain an environment for quality excellence conducive to full participation and personal and organizational growth.

This section begins by exploring the company's overall plan for human resources and how these integrate into the SBP, followed by four sections all focusing on the employee. Specifically, employee involvement, training and education, performance and recognition, and well-being and satisfaction are examined. In addition, the latter four sections are all results oriented. The examiner will want to know what is being done to and with the employee and, very importantly, how it is working out. And so once again, collection of data and documentation of these activities are necessary. Trending analysis is also required, and so collation and presentation of the data over time to show trends in things like turnover and absenteeism are important.

The initial section on overall plans should show that the company perceives the employee as integral to getting a process done. Recall from the fishbone diagram that one of the six classical system components is the personnel component. In addition, it is axiomatic that the more personnel involved in a process, the more inherent variability. These are called people-intensive processes, and the Baldrige criteria call for robust design where appropriate. It is most appropriate in people-intensive processes. Robust design calls for foolproofing, backup, redundancy, and system design that anticipates special-cause variation, identified perhaps by FMEA, and guards against it.

A TQM operation will also view people as a key ingredient of the overall process and, to that end, the number and types of personnel should match the requirements of the SBP. This section further recognizes that employees are human as opposed to other process components, and consequently, need a career path, training and education, involvement, and rewards for work well done.

All serious competitors for the Baldrige award offer job-related training, but the examiner looks for a coherence in the training efforts that relate to the company direction and that address key components of the operational plans. One company I reviewed, paid, on successful course completion, for any academic effort of their employees whether job related or not. This relates to the overall component of job enrichment and is a value-added benefit well received by employee and reviewer as well. Many excellent companies are forming relationships with local schools, whether colleges, high schools, or vocational institutions, and are bringing certain offerings into the workplace.

This is also an appropriate place to mention the types of teams that are used in the lab and the hospital. These would include the process improvement teams, the longer-term quality circle types, cross-functional teams with lab members, and other group activities used for process design, analysis, deployment, and improvement. Again, coordination of these efforts with the direction of the operation would be appropriate. For instance, if the hospital operation supports point-of-care testing, other remote testing centers, outpatient services, health fairs, wellness centers, and the like, lab support plans, operations, analysis, and improvement efforts are fitting.

In terms of involvement, reverse reviews are reported as being particularly rewarding and helpful. This is the bottom-up review as opposed to the traditional top-down process. For those companies with a fixation on sharing financials with top management as an incentive to do better, TQM companies will, in contrast, share an abbreviated financial with all levels of employees. Nothing is hidden in this area. Also all employees will be on salary, other than those required to be on hourly by law. The purpose of all of this is to break down the barriers created by the haves and have-nots, the in group and the outsiders, the privileged few and the constrained many. As mentioned at the beginning, this is a results-oriented section, and the effectiveness of these policies as well as the overall environment must be measured, the results must be analyzed, and the plans must be instituted for improvement.

This is a very rich and rewarding section if addressed sufficiently well. This category more than any other really reflects the company commitment to TQM. If the examiner sees the traditional annual employee review tied to raises with a yearly company picnic and holiday party, then the examiner has been provided with a clear window into the company's soul, and what follows must be very good to compensate for the shortcomings in this section. This isn't meant to be overly judgmental. But at this stage of the MBNQA evolution, there are companies which are repackaging traditional operations to more nearly meet the MBNQA criteria, and these can be artfully enough done to score pretty well in some of the other categories, but this one stands out. Some companies are straightforward enough to admit this and to concede that there are areas to be improved in their own evolution on the road to quality. Their artless sincerity in this regard is well received, and the well wishes of the reviewers go with them along with mutual anticipation of future efforts.

Management of Process Quality (5.0)

The management of process quality category examines the systematic processes the company uses to pursue ever higher quality and company operational performance. Examined are the key elements of process management, including research and development, design, management of process quality for all work units and suppliers, systematic quality improvement, and quality assessment.

There are five sections under this category. They begin with the design of quality services, move into the process management and internal support of the process design, explore supplier quality, a major external component of process support, and conclude with a section on evaluating how well all these things are working.

In the first section regarding the design and introduction of new lab services, the expectations would first be to see the new services formally linked both to customer requirements and the hospital mission. This would require prior identification of the customers and a knowledge of the customer key service requirements. This is a major project requiring a great deal of effort, since it requires the identification of all internal and external customers. The mission of the hospital would also have to be integrated with the new services through policy management so that the lab priorities are coordinated with management and resource support. This is the planning part of the PDCA cycle.

In the next section on management of service production and delivery, the examiner looks for an integration of the operational component with the design component. This is the do part of the PDCA cycle. The examiner also looks for a monitoring of the ongoing service processes, so that the process capability can be determined where possible and monitored for capability. In addition, when special-cause variation is noted, this section calls for a standardized method for root cause analysis. The MBNQA requires that a good plan for root cause analysis be in place and shown clearly here. This fits nicely with the quality assurance requirements of CLIA '88, which also call for remediation when things don't go quite right. And all of this also fits in nicely with the check part of the PDCA Deming wheel which is the basis for process improvement.

The next section repeats the one just reviewed, but with an emphasis on business processes and support services. If the lab is being marketed externally to the hospital, then the business processes of marketing and sales will be important. Associated with this, but also independent of external operations, is public relations, an important aspect to be addressed here. Support services include finance and accounting, computer and information services, facilities and plant management support, personnel, and secretarial and administrative support. All of the systems, by means of which the lab interacts with these ancillary departments and functions, should be clearly shown, process owners ascribed, monitoring means installed, and process improvement methods developed as priorities are assigned.

The subsequent section on supplier quality asks that the lab document means by which its quality requirements are made known to outside suppliers. Fortunately, in the lab equipment and reagent supply business, suppliers are very active in the quality movement, and this area should evolve in a mutually beneficial way. One of the components to a successful showing in this area is JIT operation. The concept of JIT operations is that a business should only inventory an amount of supplies that it needs over a short period. If the business stocks too much material, it ties up money which could be better used elsewhere, could be invested, or could just collect interest. JIT efforts have to be carefully done so as not to exhaust supplies by not accommodating unexpected demands.

The final section asks that the systems which are used for the review of data, and the integration of these data into process and overall service improvement, be shown and explained how they lead to action and improvement. The section only asks for the plans and systems which result in the data collection by monitoring the activities. It does not ask for results of the activities. The results are detailed in response to the requirements of the next category.

Quality and Operational Results (6.0)

The quality and operational results category examines the company's quality levels and improvement trends in quality, company operational performance, and supplier quality. Also examined are current quality and operational performance levels relative to those of competitors.

The summary quote from the MBNQA booklet describes this section completely. All four sections under this category are divided into only two subsections. They ask the twin questions, "How well did you do?" and "How well did you do compared to industry standards and world-class standards?" Benchmarking was mentioned in Section 2.0. Here, process improvements, in order to result in improvement in competitive position, must be better than the industry average. If a company has no improvement going on, it will fall behind the industry. Improvements which are only as good as the industry average are the minimum necessary to keep the company in business. Juran has an interesting perspective on the type and frequency of process improvements viewed collectively. He says that in going from where you are to where you want to be, the more process improvement activities going on, the steeper the slope of the cumulative improvement curve. This is shown in Figure 8.4 in which Company B has more activity going on than Company A. Consequently B is improving faster than A. It goes without saying that in order for the overall effort to be viewed as progress, the activities have to be carefully chosen and prioritized to reflect customer preferences.

The lab industry needs to collect and share data on common processes, so that laboratorians can have an idea of what industry standards are. In addition to this comparison, however, the Baldrige position would be that the lab should compare itself to world-class industries in areas in which they share a common component. For instance, Disney is frequently used as a benchmark in the general service sector. Ask yourself, "Would people rather go to my hospital or to the Magic Kingdom?" Reflect that Disney handles people really well and how could it hurt that the hospital does the same?

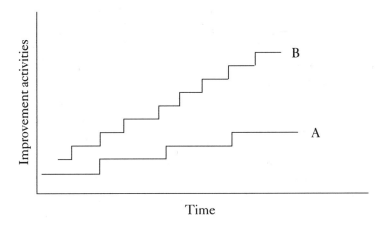

Figure 8.4: Company improvement with time.

Customer Focus and Satisfaction (7.0)

The customer focus and satisfaction category examines the company's relationships with customers and its knowledge of customer requirements and of the key quality factors that drive marketplace competitiveness. Also examined are the company's methods to determine customer satisfaction, current trends and levels of customer satisfaction and retention, and these results relative to competitors.

The Baldrige position is that pleasing customers is good. In this, it reflects standard TQM thinking. This category is a complete section which isolates the company planning, operations, process evaluation, and results exclusively as they relate to the external customer. The initial section asks how the lab assesses current and future requirements of customers. In this, the criteria consider the market as a moving target, and that although the current situation may be a good one, with the passage of time, continual improvement must be tied closely to changing customer requirements. The lab's external customers, with the exception of the regulatory folks, will actually be internal to the hospital (nursing, ER, surgery, the units, physicians, and so on), and a formal means for continually assessing and prioritizing their views is required. One way of doing this is by using quality function deployment. QFD is a matrix technique which can do this, but it is not easy. At least a controlled operation should be in place which includes continual assessment of the customers' views through phone and written surveys, checklists, and evaluation of data by teams addressing process improvement or cross-functional issues which may be identified through these assessments.

Following this, criteria must be developed which will reflect customer relationship management. In other words, the prior section shows the planning function of the PDCA cycle, and the next two center on the do part, or operations. Customer relationship management and customer commitment show the means by, and degree to which, the lab pledge to customer satisfaction is carried out. Under this heading is a section on customer service personnel and their selection, training, development, and career path opportunities.

In the final section on the results of the customer satisfaction operations, the now-familiar request is made for illustrations showing how well the company compares to industry and world-class standards. This is to be shown in a trending format so that progress with time can be assessed.

Summary

A quality management program may be structured around the Baldrige criteria. These sections give a cursory review of the MBNQA criteria as they relate to a hospital lab operation. To get a copy of the MBNQA criteria, write to MBNQA/NIST, Route 270 and Quince Orchard Road, Administration Building, Room A537, Gaithersburg, Maryland 20899; 301-975-2036, Fax 301-948-3716.

NOTES

1. CDRH-FDA Guideline on General Principles of Process Validation, May 1987. Division of Manufacturing and Product Quality, HFM-320, Office of Compliance.

2. See Note 1.

3. Berwick, D. M., A. B. Godfrey, and J. Roessner. *Curing Health Care: New Strategies for Quality Improvement.* San Francisco: Jossey-Bass, 1990.

Appendix A:
Format for Procedures

In writing procedures for laboratory use, it is helpful to have a descriptive format. The format mandates an architecture for the procedure and a structure which lends itself to a thorough and complete description of the process. Having the format acts as a check sheet so that all characteristics of one procedure are reflected in all procedures. Basically the format rests on the five W's and one H (where, why, when, what, who, and how).

It is traditional to view a procedure as a set of instructions on how to do a process, but it also has to include who is responsible, when they do each step, why the procedure is necessary, what are the required components—either by equipment, reagents, or special materials—and when to do steps, or the timing.

In addition, each procedure should have a flowchart of the process it describes. Some procedures are lengthy and don't lend themselves to a manageable flowchart. In this case, the procedure could be broken up into components for clarity and ease of understanding. When this is done, the main reference procedure acts as an umbrella under which the component procedures are referenced.

This format is meant as an example of a general procedural format. Those interested in more detail on technical procedures are referred to the NCCLS document GP2-A2, "Clinical Laboratory Technical Procedure Manuals," 2d ed., July 1992. Available from NCCLS, 771 E. Lancaster Avenue, Villanova, Pennsylvania 19085.

	No. 001	Rev. 0
General operating procedure	Page 1	of 5
	Issued by:	
Title: Format for procedures	Date:	

1.0. Purpose and Scope

The purpose of this procedure is to delineate the form which internal standard operating procedures shall take. Its scope extends to all procedures which the lab employs, whether technical or operational.

2.0. Responsibility

It is the responsibility of all individuals who write procedures at this facility to comply with these directives.

3.0. Precautions and Safety Directives

3.1. Write clearly and simply. Draft the procedure in a way which can be easily understood.

3.2. Define all parameters and procedural steps. Leave nothing to the imagination.

4.0. References

Use 42 CFR 493.1211 and 42 CFR 493.1701. These two sections of the Code of Federal Regulations are portions of the regulation commonly referred to as the Clinical Laboratory Improvement Act of 1988. Specifically, they address the requirements for a written procedure manual and a written quality assurance program.

General operating procedure	No. 001	Rev. 0
	Page 2 of 5	
Title: Format for procedures	Issued by:	
	Date:	

5.0. Procedure

5.1. Title and Headers

The procedure shall have a header, to appear on each page. This is the what of the five W's and one H. The header is to appear on each page and should contain the following:

    a. The title of the procedure.
    b. The control number (unique numerical identification) of the procedure.
    c. The date the procedure was issued.
    d. A signature of the issuing individual.
    e. The revision number of the procedure. These are expressed as Rev. 0, 1, 2, 3, and so on.
    f. The page number. As an example, this is to be expressed as "page 2 of 3." List the page number and the total number of pages in the SOP.

5.2. Review Schedule

The procedure shall have room to indicate when the next review is scheduled. It shall also reflect the latest review by signature and date.

5.3. Procedure Flowchart

The procedure shall have appended a flowchart which outlines the procedure in detail sufficient to enable process improvement and critique (FMEA, FTA) to be done using the flowchart as a basis.

	No. 001 Rev. 0
General operating procedure	Page 3 of 5
	Issued by:
Title: Format for procedures	Date:

5.4. Procedure Organization

The procedure should be organized as follows:

5.4.1. Section 1, Purpose and Scope. This is the why section and addresses the intent of the SOP and the areas where it applies.

5.4.2. Section 2, Responsibility. This is the who section. Specifically, the process ownership should be established here.

5.4.3. Section 3, Precautions. Both safety concerns and general caveats are addressed here. This, as well as Section 5, address the how, where, and when of the procedure.

5.4.4. Section 4, References. List both technical references, such as inserts, and regulatory references, such as CLIA, FDA, Medicare, State, OSHA, and so on.

5.4.5. Section 5, Procedure. Usually, this is the lengthiest section and includes the stepwise, detailed process description. For analytical procedures it will include specimen collection as well as the analytical steps. For a general operations procedure it will be the last section. The following sections are for analytical procedures requiring instrumental measurement and reporting of results.

5.4.6. Section 6, Quality Control. Detail the number and types of control materials and the periodicity of their use. Mention charting techniques and requirements for run rejection or review.

General operating procedure	No. 001 Rev. 0
	Page 4 of 5
Title: Format for procedures	Issued by:
	Date:

5.4.7. Section 7, Instrument Maintenance. If an instrument is used in the technique, detail the preventive maintenance schedule and also the source of emergency maintenance. Also describe back-up techniques if the instrument is expected to be down for a lengthy period.

5.4.8. Section 8, Reporting. Describe how the reporting function is done from the instrument readout through transfer to the report distribution group. Include a description of supervisory review and any other quality checks necessary prior to release of the report.

5.5. Routing

Circulate the completed procedure through the established concurrence routing. When all involved section heads have signed off, issue the procedure.

5.6. Procedure Issue

Issue the new procedure to document control, the archive section, and all involved departments. Collect the outdated procedure, verify that the outdated procedure is archived, and destroy all other copies of the outdated procedure.

General operating procedure	No. 001 Rev. 0
	Page 5 of 5
Title: Format for procedures	Issued by:
	Date:

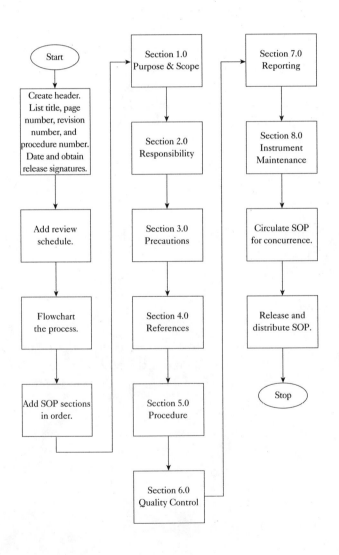

Appendix B:
The Quality
Assurance Program,
CLIA '88

Based on the format suggested in Appendix A, the following is given as an example of a nontechnical procedure. Readers may find this useful in their own laboratory settings.

The Clinical Laboratory Improvement Act of 1967 (CLIA '67) required that laboratories doing business in interstate commerce have a quality assurance program. The requirement did not specify that the procedure be written. Since a companion section in the regulations required a written procedure manual, the regulation was satisfied by defaulting to these procedures as encompassing the requirements of the QA program.

In March 14, 1990, the combined regulations were written which continued to focus on previously regulated labs, but combined Medicare and interstate regulations. The section on quality assurance remained the same, and inspectors were given the option of inspecting under this set or the older CLIA '67 set of regulations.

Then, in 1992, after four years of deliberation, CLIA '88 was issued and the section on QA contained the words *written procedure*. Section 42 CFR 493.1701 reads, "Each laboratory performing moderate or high complexity testing, or both, must establish and follow written policies and procedures for a comprehensive quality assurance program."

The specification goes on to state that the quality of the total testing process (preanalytic, analytic, and postanalytic) must be monitored and evaluated. In essence, the regulators are viewing the lab as a three-part system. The subsequent sections delineate the components of each of these three parts, as well as an extra-analytic component having to do with external evaluation, complaint handling, and the audit function.

One way of meeting this standard is to design a quality assurance SOP built specifically around the stated objectives of the regulation. In essence, the SOP should reflect the regulation exactly so there is no doubt that each and every element of the regulation is specifically addressed.

Under the responsibility section of the SOP, a quality assurance committee is referenced which has the charter requirement of reviewing the regulatory standards on a periodic basis. That the requirements are addressed during this interval is controlled by a check sheet which is part of the SOP and summarizes the standard requirements. This procedure, modeled after the prior SOP "Format for Procedures," (Appendix A) is as shown.

General operating procedure	No. 002	Rev. 0
	Page 1	of 5
Title:	Issued by:	
Quality assurance program	Date:	

1.0. Purpose and Scope

The purpose of this procedure is to delineate the laboratory responsibility under the CLIA '88 regulatory requirements for a written quality assurance program. Its scope extends to the analytical component as well as pre- and postanalytic processes.

2.0. Responsibility

The laboratory has in place a quality assurance committee, chaired by the director, which may meet as frequently as needed, but minimally on a quarterly basis, to evaluate the effectiveness of the laboratory's procedures and policies as mandated under 42 CFR 493.1701 and the following.

The purpose of the committee is to evaluate the effectiveness of the laboratory's policies, identify and correct problems, assure the accuracy and timely reporting of test results, and assure the adequacy and competency of the staff. In addition, the committee will review and summarize activities of the quality action teams.

As necessary, this group will revise procedures based on the results of these evaluations. The laboratory must meet the standards of Subpart P as clarified below, specifically with regard to the lab services offered, the complexity of testing performed and reported, and the unique practices of each testing entity. All proceedings of this committee as they relate to quality assurance activities must be documented.

Quality action teams will be assigned by the committee to monitor ongoing activities in the areas identified by this regulation.

General operating procedure	No. 002 Rev. 0
	Page 2 of 5
	Issued by:
Title: Quality assurance program	Date:

3.0. Precautions and Safety Directives

All sections of CLIA '88 referenced below shall be specifically addressed.

4.0. References

    a. 42 CFR 493, Subpart P, "Quality Assurance for Moderate or High Complexity Testing," or both. Sections 1701, 1703, 1705, 1707, 1709, 1711, 1713, 1715, 1717, 1719, 1721 (CLIA '88, section on quality assurance).

    b. Check sheet 002-CS.

5.0. Procedure

    5.1. Preanalytic Testing Standards

        5.1.1. Patient preparation, specimen collection, labeling, preservation, and transportation

        5.1.2. The laboratory test requisition requirements

        5.1.3. The criteria used for specimen rejection

        5.1.4. The organization of the test report forms

        5.1.5. The timely reporting of test results based on testing priorities such as stat and routine

        5.1.6. The accuracy and reliability of the test reporting systems as well as requirements for storage and retrieval of test results

	No. 002 Rev. 0
General operating procedure	Page 3 of 5
	Issued by:
Title: Quality assurance program	Date:

5.2. Analytical Component Standards

5.2.1. Analytical processes as follows:

a. The evaluation of calibration and control data for each test method
b. The evaluation of patient test results used to verify test reference ranges
c. Errors in reported test results

5.2.2. Proficiency testing review and assessment, including remediation associated with unsuccessful performance

5.2.3. Comparison of instrument performance addressing paired testing of instruments either using different methodologies or at different sites. This function must be performed at least twice a year.

5.2.3.1. If the laboratory performs assays for analytes not included under Subpart I (Proficiency Testing), it must verify the accuracy and reliability of these at least twice a year.

5.3. The Postanalytical Component

5.3.1. The relationship of clinical information to test results is reviewed with the following criteria in mind.

a. Patient age
b. Patient sex

	No. 002 Rev. 0
General operating procedure	Page 4 of 5
	Issued by:
Title: Quality assurance program	Date:

     c. Patient diagnosis or pertinent clinical data
     d. The distribution of patient test results
     e. Relationship of the patient test results to other test parameters

5.3.2. Personnel Assessment

The effectiveness of the laboratory's ongoing policies and procedures for assuring employee competence, or the competence of other laboratory employees such as consultants, is also reviewed.

5.3.3. Communications

The committee reviews, confirms, and documents all calls from accounts which relate to either pre- or postanalytical communications problems between the lab and the account.

5.3.4. Complaint Investigation

The committee investigates any complaint which is received by the laboratory. It also reflects any remediation accompanying the investigation.

General operating procedure	No. 002	Rev. 0
	Page 5 of 5	
Title: Quality assurance program	Issued by:	
	Date:	

5.3.5. Quality Assurance Review

The laboratory committee reviews the problems identified, and subsequently reviews them with the laboratory staff. System improvements installed as a result of problem solving are also reviewed with the staff. The process is documented in the weekly lab meeting minutes.

5.3.6. Quality Assurance Records

5.3.6.1. All records of quality assurance activities are maintained in the laboratory for a period of two years following the last use of the procedure. All records are available for HHS inspection.

5.3.6.2. The records are maintained attached to the check sheet (002-CS) documenting the monthly meeting.

	No. 002-cs Rev. 0
General operating procedure	Page 1 of 3
	Issued by:
Title: Q. A. program—Check Sheet	Date:

Date: _____

Attendance: _____ _____

_____ _____

_____ _____

5.0 Check Items

   5.1 Preanalytic Testing Standards

      5.1.1. Patient preparation, specimen collection, labeling, preserva-
             tion, and transportation
      5.1.2. The laboratory test requisition requirements
      5.1.3. The criteria used for specimen rejection
      5.1.4. The organization of the test report forms
      5.1.5. The timely reporting of test results based on testing priori-
             ties such as stat and routine
      5.1.6. The accuracy and reliability of the test reporting systems as
             well as requirements for storage and retrieval of test results
   5.2. Analytical Component Standards

      5.2.1. Analytical processes as follows:

         a. The evaluation of calibration and control data for each
            test method
         b. The evaluation of patient test results used to verify test
            reference ranges
         c. Errors in reported test results

      5.2.2. Proficiency testing review and assessment, including reme-
             diation associated with unsuccessful performance
      5.2.3. Comparison of instrument performance addressing paired

	No. 002-cs Rev. 0
General operating procedure	Page 2 of 3
	Issued by:
Title: Q. A. program—Check Sheet	Date:

testing of instruments either using different methodologies, or at different sites. This function must be performed at least twice a year.

5.2.3.1. Reliability and accuracy of analytes not covered under Subpart I (Proficiency Testing) are also validated twice a year.

5.3. The Postanalytical Component

5.3.1. The relationship of clinical information to test results is reviewed with the following criteria in mind.

 a. Patient age
 b. Patient sex
 c. Patient diagnosis or pertinent clinical data
 d. The distribution of patient test results
 e. Relationship of the patient test results to other test parameters

5.3.2. Personnel Assessment

The effectiveness of the laboratory's ongoing policies and procedures for assuring employee competence, or the competence of other laboratory employees such as consultants, is also reviewed.

5.3.3. Communications

The committee reviews, confirms, and documents all calls from accounts which relate to either pre- or postanalytical communications problems between the lab and the account.

	No. 002-cs Rev. 0
General operating procedure	Page 3 of 3
	Issued by:
Title: Q. A. program—Check Sheet	Date:

5.3.4. Complaint Investigation

The committee investigates any complaint which is received by the laboratory. It also reflects any remediation accompanying the investigation.

5.3.5. Quality Assurance Review

The laboratory committee reviews problems identified, and subsequently reviews them with the laboratory staff. System improvements installed as a result of problem solving are also reviewed with the staff. The process is documented in the lab staff meeting minutes.

5.3.6. Quality Assurance Records

5.3.6.1. All records of quality assurance activities are maintained in the laboratory for a period of two years following the last use of the procedure. All records are available for HHS inspection.

5.3.6.2. I certify that the above listed items were reviewed during the meeting which occurred this date and any support or reference documentation is attached to this form. The documentation summarizes the minutes of the meeting as well as any action taken, subcommittee activity begun, or remedial activity either in process or completed.

Signed: _____ _____

(Laboratory Director)   (Date)

Appendix C:
Glossary of Acronyms

ASQC

The American Society for Quality Control. The premier professional quality organization in the United States, located in Milwaukee, Wisconsin.

ATF

The Bureau of Alcohol, Tobacco and Firearms. Regulates the use of lab alcohol.

CBER

Center for Biological Evaluation and Research. A division of the FDA regulating the blood and plasma collection industry and biological kits and components.

CDC

The Centers for Disease Control in Atlanta, Georgia. Responsible with HCFA for setting complexity levels for testing regulated under CLIA '88.

CDRH

Center for Devices and Radiological Health. A division of the FDA regulating medical device manufacturers.

CLIA '88

The Clinical Laboratory Improvement Act of 1988. A set of regulations designed to place all clinical laboratories under one set of standards. Deployed by HCFA.

CPM

Critical Path Method. Developed by E. I. du Pont de Nemours & Co., this method of project tracking allows for project compression with increased funding.

CQE

Certified quality engineer. A professional certification administered by ASQC which requires qualification by education and experience, passing a six-hour examination, and continuing education for recertification. The society also administers the certified quality auditor (CQA), the certified reliability engineer (CRE), and the quality engineer in training (QEIT).

DEA

Drug Enforcement Agency. Regulates standards used in toxicology laboratories and certain lab buffers.

DERM

Department of Environmental Regulation and Management. Local environmental regulatory groups sometimes called DERC (C = Control).

DRGs

Diagnosis related groups.

EMEA

Error mode and effect analysis. A variant of FMEA which concentrates solely on processes which have people as part of the system and the potential human error component.

EPA

Environmental Protection Agency. Regulates the lab with respect to its waste streams.

FDA

The U.S. Food and Drug Administration. Regulates blood banks and blood diagnostic kits under CBER and medical device manufacturers under CDRH.

FMEA

Failure mode and effect analysis. A technique used to assess potential process performance prospectively.

FPL

Florida Power & Light. Headquartered in Miami, the only overseas company ever to win the Deming Prize, Japan's principal quality award.

FTA

Fault tree analysis. A technique used to assess process performance retrospectively.

GANTT or Gantt Chart

Sometimes used as the verb *to Gantt*. A formal way of visually representing a project.

GMP

Also called cGMP for current Good Manufacturing Practice. An FDA minimum performance criterion for lab suppliers and manufacturers.

HCFA

Health Care Finance Administration. Under HHS, administers CLIA '88 and the Medicare program.

HHS

The department of Health and Human Services, run by a cabinet-level appointee. CDC, NIH, HCFA, and FDA report to this department.

JCAHO

Joint Commission on Accreditation of Healthcare Organizations.

JIT

Just-in-time. A supply purchasing-and-delivery system that results in appropriate levels of inventory matched to service and product delivery requirements. Results in minimal cash outlay for stored supplies and materials.

JUSE

The Union of Japanese Scientists and Engineers. A Japanese professional business society.

LPC

Least preferred co-worker. A contingency management test designed by Fred Fiedler.

MBO

Management by objective. Management system popularized by Peter Drucker.

MLO

Medical Laboratory Observer in Montvale, New Jersey.

MBNQA

Malcolm Baldrige National Quality Award. The premier U.S. quality award administered by NIST.

MBP

Management by policy. The western equivalent of the Japanese TQC management system called hoshin kanri.

MTBF

Mean time between failures. A statistically derived expression of product reliability.

NCCLS

National Committee for Clinical Laboratory Standards. Operates a consensus mechanism among professionals in health care practice, government, and industry for the development of national and international voluntary standards.

NCEP

National Cholesterol Education Program. One of only two national health programs launched by the NIH. The other was the High Blood Pressure Awareness Program.

NIDA

National Institute for Drug Abuse. Regulates and qualifies toxicology laboratories.

NIH

The National Institutes for Health. In Washington, D.C., the NIH consist of seven separate institutes for research into human diseases.

NIST

National Institute for Standards and Technology. Formerly the National Bureau of Standards, this institute, under the Department of Commerce, administers the Malcolm Baldrige National Quality Award in conjunction with ASQC.

NRC

Nuclear Regulatory Commission. Regulates the use of radionuclides and the disposal of radioactive waste in labs exceeding *de minimus* usage.

OR

Operations research. Same as management science, uses qualitative and statistical tools for management planning.

OSHA

Occupational Safety and Health Administration. Regulates the lab's hazard control, specifically blood-borne pathogens and chemicals. Also requires an overall safe workplace.

PDCA

Plan, Do, Check, Act. Developed by Walter A. Shewhart and frequently called the Deming wheel, has evolved into the basis for process improvement.

PDPC

Process decision program chart. A formal method for process improvement which combines aspects of FTA, FMEA, and contingency planning.

PERT

Program evaluation review technique. A project tracking technique used for the *Polaris* submarine. Amenable to statistical OR techniques.

POL

Physician's office lab.

QAT

Quality action team.

QC Story
A formal means by which system improvement processes are documented.

QFD
Quality function deployment. A Japanese technique for integrating customers' quality perceptions into process improvement planning by means of a specialized matrix.

QIDW
Quality in everyday work. Also called quality in everyday operations, refers to TQM deployment and use at the line level of operations.

SBP
Strategic business plan. Formalism by means of which the company mission and vision are linked to short-term and long-range operational plans commensurate with financial capabilities and projections.

SDCA
Standardize, Do, Check, Act. Before a process can be improved by PDCA techniques, it must be standardized to remove special-cause variation so that it is in statistical control.

SPC
Statistical process control. Introduced by Walter A. Shewhart as a formal way of assessing process performance and tracking improvement.

TAT
Turnaround time. An overall measure of lab response from request to report.

TQC
Total quality control. A term introduced by Armand V. Feigenbaum which the Japanese liked. They used it to characterize their own quality efforts. In this book and in much western literature, TQC refers to the Japanese quality movement.

TQM

Total quality management. A term used to refer to the western and U.S. version of the quality movement.

USDA

U.S. Department of Agriculture. Regulates lab use of animals.

ZD

Zero defects. Originally associated with World War II quality efforts, is now more frequently associated with a management program developed by Philip Crosby.

Index